Learning Imaging

Series Editors:

R. Ribes · A. Luna · P. Ros

R. Ribes · P. Kuschnir · A. Luna
J. C. Vilanova · J. M. Jimenez-Hoyuela
(Eds.)

Learning Cardiac Imaging

Springer

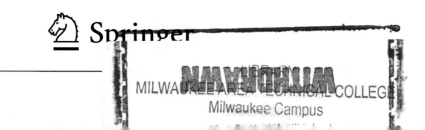
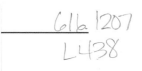

Ramón Ribes MD PhD
Reina Sofia University Hospital
14005 Córdoba
Spain
ribesb@gmail.com

Paola Kuschnir MD
Centro de Diagnóstico Enrique Rossi
2777 Buenos Aires
Argentina
paolakus@fibertel.com.ar

Antonio Luna MD
Clinica Las Nieves Sercosa
Carmelo Torres, 2
23007 Jaén
Spain
aluna70@sercosa.com

Joan C. Vilanova
Department of Magnetic Resonance
Clinica Girona
Lorenzana, 36
17002 Girona
Spain
kvilanova@comg.es

José Manuel Jimenez-Hoyuela MD PhD
Hospital Regional Universitario
Carlos Haya
Servicio de Medicina Nuclear
Avenida Carlos Haya, s/n
29010 Málaga
Spain
josem.jimenezhoyuela.sspa@juntadeandalucia.es

ISBN: 978-3-540-79082-2   e-ISBN: 978-3-540-79084-6

DOI: 10.1007/978-3-540-79084-6

Springer Heidelberg Dordrecht London New York

Library of Congress Control Number: 2009931694

Cover design: eStudioCalamar, Figueres/Berlin

Printed on acid-free paper

9 8 7 6 5 4 3 2 1

Springer is part of Springer Science+Business Media (www.springer.com)

"To Anabel Ribes Bautista
for her always sensible advice."

RAMÓN RIBES

"To all my
teachers and *colleagues*
who I deeply admire and appreciate.
To my *parents*, my *husband*,
and *daughter*, who enrich my *life*."

PAOLA KUSCHNIR

"To my Marias"

ANTONIO LUNA

"To my wife *Cris* and my children
Cristina and *Eduard* for their love
and for accommodating the sacrifices of
personal time."

JOAN C. VILANOVA

"To my *Parents* and my wife."

JOSE MANUEL JIMENEZ-HOYUELA

Preface

After the publication of *Learning Diagnostic Imaging*, which was an introductory teaching file to the ten radiological subspecialties included in the American Boards of Radiology, we began to write a series of teaching files on each radiological subspecialty.

If the first book of the series was mainly aimed at residents and provided them with an introductory tool to the study of radiology, the subsequent volumes of the series try to provide the reader with an introduction to the study of each radiological subspecialty.

In *Learning Cardiac Imaging*, we intend to review cardiac imaging from the perspective of the six imaging modalities usually performed to obtain anatomic and functional information of the heart.

In old days, conventional radiographs gave us some information about the anatomy and, only secondarily, the pathophysiology of the heart. With the advent of echocardiography, the heart could be studied dynamically. Nuclear Medicine and Cardiac MR allowed the study of cardiac function. 32- and 64-detector multislice CT let us obtain images of the coronary tree in a noninvasive approach.

Cardiac imaging is complex and many health care professionals are needed, firstly, in the obtention and, secondly, in the interpretation of the images. Not only radiolologists, cardiologists, and nuclear medicine physicians are needed, specialized nurses and technicians are indispensable to obtain diagnostic images of such a dynamic anatomic structure as the heart.

The authorship of the book reflects its multidisciplinary approach of the book. Only the cooperation of radiologists, cardiologists, and nuclear medicine physicians has made this book possible.

The multiplicity of imaging modalities currently performed in the study of the heart – conventional radiology, conventional angiography, echocardiography, multislice CT, magnetic resonance, and nuclear medicine – is one of the most distinguishing features of cardiac imaging and it makes it one of the most attractive areas of the radiological knowledge.

Córdoba, Spain, September 10, 2009   RAMÓN RIBES

Contents

3 Cardiac Magnetic Resonance

Joan C. Vilanova, Antonio Luna, Manel Morales, Xavier Albert,
Joaquim Barceló, and Ramón Ribes

4 Nuclear Cardiology

José Manuel Jiménez-Hoyuela García
Simeón Ortega Lozano, Dolores Martínez del Valle Torres,
Antonio Guitiérrez Cardo, and Esperanza Ramos Moreno

Contributing Authors

Xavier Albert
Department of Magnetic Resonance
Clínica Girona
Girona
Spain

Gustavo Avegliano
Cardiac Imaging Department
Instituto Cardiovascular de Buenos Aires
Buenos Aires, Argentina
Research Group for Computational Imaging &
Simulation Technologies in Biomedicine (CISTIB)
Department of Information and Communication
Technologies, Universitat Pompeu Fabra
Barcelona
Spain

Joaquim Barceló
Department of Magnetic Resonance
Clínica Girona
Girona
Spain

Antonio Guitiérrez Cardo
Servicio de Medicina Nuclear
Hospital Regional Universitario
Málaga
Spain

José Manuel Jiménez-Hoyuela García
Servicio de Medicina Nuclear
Hospital Regional Universitario
Málaga
Spain

Antonio Luna
Department of Magnetic Resonance
Clínica Las Nieves
Jaén
Spain

Dolores Martínez del Valle Torres
Servicio de Medicina Nuclear
Hospital Regional Universitario
Málaga
Spain

Manel Morales
Department of Magnetic Resonance
Clínica Girona
Girona
Spain

Simeón Ortega Lozano
Servicio de Medicina Nuclear
Hospital Regional Universitario
Málaga
Spain

Lucio T. Padilla
Centro de Diagnostico Dr. E. Rossi
Cardiac Imaging Department
Instituto Cardiovascular de Buenos Aires
Buenos Aires University
Buenos Aires
Argentina

Esperanza Ramos Moreno
Servicio de Medicina Nuclear
Hospital Regional Universitario
Málaga
Spain

RAMÓN RIBES
Interventional Radiology and MR Units
Reina Sofía University Hospital
Córdoba
Spain

RICARDO RONDEROS
Cardiac Imaging Department
Instituto Cardiovascular de Buenos Aires
Buenos Aires,
Argentina

SANTIAGO ROSSI
Centro de Diagnostico Dr. E. Rossi
Buenos Aires, Argentina
Radiology, Favaloro University
Buenos Aires
Argentina

M. AGUSTINA SCIANCALEPORE
Centro de Diagnostico Dr. E. Rossi
Cardiac Imaging Department
Instituto Cardiovascular de Buenos Aires
Buenos Aires
Argentina

MARCELO TRIVI
Cardiac Imaging Department
Instituto Cardiovascular de Buenos Aires
Buenos Aires
Argentina

JOAN C. VILANOVA
Department of Magnetic Resonance
Clínica Girona
Girona
Spain

Introduction

X. Lucaya

Cardiac imaging has come a long way. Currently, excellent diagnostic images of most cardiac malformations can be obtained by US, MSCT, MRI or nuclear medicine.

Despite the many advantages of modern technology, it should be remembered that, not so long ago, we were able to obtain significant information by a careful examination of plain films. A large number of correct diagnoses could be made by combining plain film features with clinical information and EKG findings. Thus, in cyanotic babies, a right aortic arch would suggest either tetralogy of Fallot or truncus arteriosus. While the former usually presents with decreased pulmonary vascularity and normal-sized heart, the latter presents with cardiomegaly and increased pulmonary circulation.

In the following sets of images we are going to pay homage to conventional radiology, the only way to see the heart in the old days.

Figure 1 shows a chest X-ray in an infant with total anomalous pulmonary venous return. In this entity, all pulmonary veins drain below the diaphragm. Affected patients will usually present with cyanosis and plain chest films will show a normal-sized heart, pulmonary venous congestion and lymphatic ectasia. Venous congestion manifests as ill-defined linear densities and lymphatic ectasia as Kerley lines. In addition to any type of obstructed total anomalous pulmonary venous return, these radiological features can also be found in patients with cor triatriatum (septated left atrium). Careful cardiac ultrasound will provide the definitive diagnosis.

Cardiomegaly and decreased pulmonary vascularity are the hallmark of Ebstein's anomaly or pulmonary artery atresia with intact ventricular septum. In Ebstein's anomaly the right cardiac border is somewhat more prominent than in pulmonary artery atresia (Fig. 2). EKG and US features play a key role in the differentiation of these two entities.

Repeated episodes of bronchitis or upper respiratory infections and/or stridor are the main clinical features in patients with vascular rings. Plain films can suggest the diagnosis, as in the case of Fig. 3. In most vascular rings, the trachea will be displaced, narrowed or indented. Barium esophagogram and, mostly, CT or MRI will confirm the diagnosis.

It is evident that new techniques play a leading role in the diagnosis of most cardiac malformations and that the diagnostic importance of plain film findings has declined significantly, to such an extent that nowadays we radiologists pay little attention to the valuable information which may occasionally be provided by the humble and inexpensive plain film, particularly when more sophisticated techniques are unavailable. Furthermore, plain film findings can influence the decision as to how to proceed and help to avoid unnecessary examinations and reduce the radiation dose to the patient.

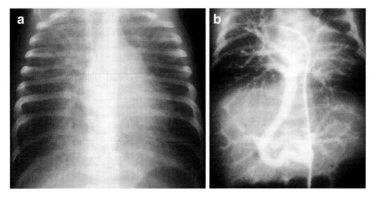

Fig. 1

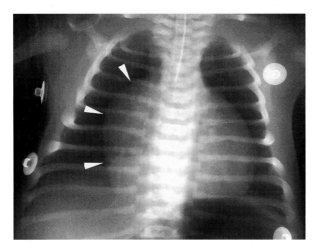

Fig. 2

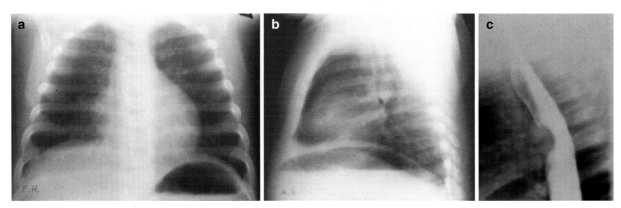

Fig. 3

Figure 1 (a, b) A 2-day-old infant with cyanosis. Chest X-ray shows a normal-sized heart and multiple bilateral linear densities corresponding to pulmonary venous congestion and/or lymphatic ectasia. These findings are very suggestive of obstructed pulmonary venous return. Cardiac catheterization confirmed the diagnosis (b). All pulmonary veins drain into a collector that runs into the portal vein.

Figure 2 A 1-week-old infant with cyanosis. Chest X-ray shows an enlarged heart with prominent right border and decreased pulmonary vascularity. These findings and the EKG features were suggestive of Ebstein's anomaly, which was confirmed by cardiac ultrasound.

Figure 3 (a, b, c) A 1-year-old infant with recurrent episodes of severe wheezing. AP chest X-ray is normal. The lateral projection shows a soft-tissue density between the trachea and the oesophagus, confirmed on the barium esophagogram. This feature suggested the diagnosis of pulmonary artery sling, which was later confirmed.

Cardiac Multislice CT

Lucio T. Padilla, M. Agustina Sciancalepore, and Santiago Rossi (Contributors)

Introduction

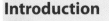

Cardiovascular disease (CVD) is the leading cause of death and disability worldwide.
- Probability at _ birth of dying from CVD is 47 vs. 22% from cancer.
- USA: 36.3% of 2.39 million deaths in 2004. One in every 36 s.
- Leading cause of hospital admissions: CAD 16% (1979–2003).
- 68% of patients who experience an MI have less than 50% stenosis at the time of the event.
- According to the American Heart Association, 62% of women and 50% of men who died suddenly of coronary heart disease had no warning from prior symptoms.

Early detection of stenosis/risk assessment in asymptomatic patients

Exclusion of CAD:
- Low- and intermediate-risk patients
- Prior to (noncardiac) surgery

Potential Applications of Computed Tomography (CT) Coronary Angiography

Detection and/or exclusion of stenosis:
- Atypical (unstable) chest pain, emergency room: triple rule out
- Inconclusive stress tests

Evaluation of congenital anomalies

Substitution of diagnostic cath

Prior to coronary intervention

High-risk patients: aortic disease

Adjuvant to coronary angiography:
- Plaque characterization
- Complicated coronary cath

Follow-up:
- Percutaneous coronary angioplasty (PTCA)
- Coronary artery bypass surgery (CABG) ~ postop complications

There is every reason to believe that over the next decade, CCTA will take on an ever-increasing role in the management of CVD.

During the last two decades CT has evolved into a powerful cardiac imaging tool. Beginning with the availability of four-slice spiral CT systems in 2000, rapid improvements in the spatial and temporal resolution of multislice CT (MSCT) have facilitated practical coronary CT angiography (CTA). With the introduction of 64-slice scanners in 2004, interest in, and clinical use of, coronary CTA increased explosively.

Case 1.1

█

Bicuspid Aortic Valve and Coronary Artery Disease

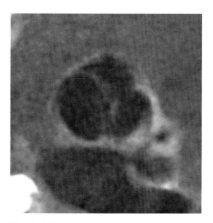

Fig. 1.1.1

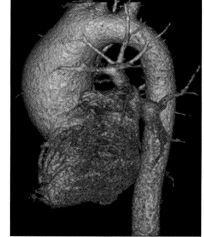

Fig. 1.1.2

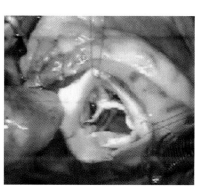

Fig. 1.1.3

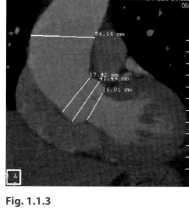

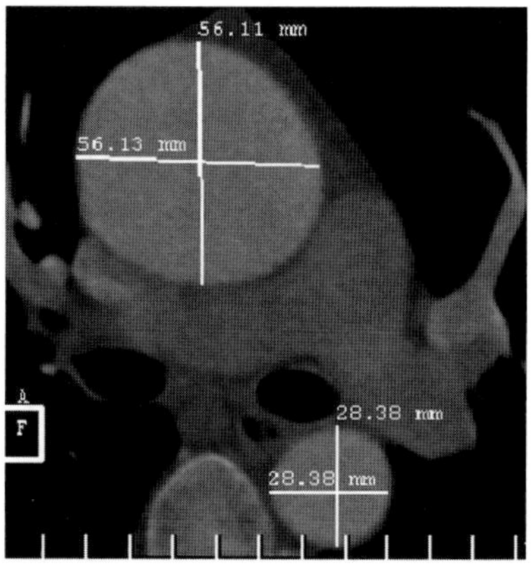

Fig. 1.1.4

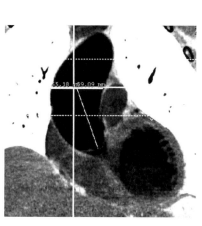

Fig. 1.1.5

Fig. 1.1.6

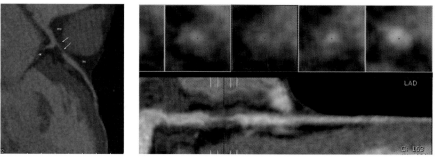

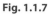

Fig. 1.1.7

Fig. 1.1.8

A 38-year-old male, smoker, family history of CAD. Complaining of chest pain during the last 2 months, NHYA II. Functional test with moderate ischemia in anterior territory. The physical examination revealed: normal blood pressure and systolic ejection murmur at the right upper sternal border that radiates to the neck. The echocardiography revealed bicuspid aortic valve (BAV), moderate aortic insufficiency and ascending aorta dilatation. MSCT was required for the assessment of aortic and coronary anatomy with the purpose of defining surgical treatment.

Comments

BAV is one of the most common isolated congenital cardiac abnormalities, present in at least 1 or 2% of the population, and predominate in men. The BAV may function normally throughout life, or it may develop progressive calcification with stenosis or regurgitation. Severe stenosis develops most often in the fifth or sixth decade.

The BAV should be considered a disease of the entire aortic root.

It is associated with accelerated degeneration of the aortic media, indicating that BAV disease is an ongoing pathological process. Inadequate production of fibrillin-1 during valvulogenesis may disrupt the formation of the aortic valve cusps, resulting in a BAV and weakened aortic root. Loss of structural support of the aorta may result in progressive aortic dilation, aneurysm formation, and dissection.

Fifty percent of young patients with a functionally normal aortic valve have echocardiography evidence of aortic dilation. Serious complications develop in 33% of patients with a BAV, so the bicuspid valve may be responsible for more deaths and morbidity than the combined effects of all other congenital heart defects. Aortic root replacement is recommended more aggressively for patients with BAV with aortic dilation than for patients with tricuspid aortic valve. For the evaluation of these patients MSCT is a method that allows functional and anatomical information of the valve, and rules out aortic dissection or other aortic complications. It also allows taking measurements that are useful for the surgeon to choose the right prosthesis and evaluate CAD.

Imaging Findings

A noninvasive coronary angiotomography was performed with a 64-row-detector CT after the intravenous administration of nonionic contrast dynamically. The coronary segmentation was established in 2D and 3D volume rendering. Aortic valve evidenced bicuspids (image finding correlated with the aortic valve seen in surgery), aortic ring had a diameter of 26.9 mm, sinotubular junction was 37.42 mm, and ascending aorta was 56 × 56 mm at the level of the pulmonary artery bifurcation. Ascending aorta dilatation rose up to the origin of the braquiocefalic trunk, at which site the aorta measured 40 mm (Figs. 1.1.1–1.1.5). The distance from the maximal opening of the valve to the maximal ascending aortic dilatation is also a useful measurement to choose the prosthesis to be used (as shown in Fig. 1.1.6). CAD was found in proximal segment of left anterior descending artery (LAD) with severe obstruction due to a soft plaque (multiplanar reconstructing and vessel analysis view in Fig. 1.1.7). No other significant CAD was found. With these findings patient underwent coronary artery bypass with a left internal mammary artery (LIMA) to LAD and aortic valve and ascending aorta replacement (Benthal de Bono surgery).

Case 1.2

■

MSCT for the Assessment of Aortic Coarctation

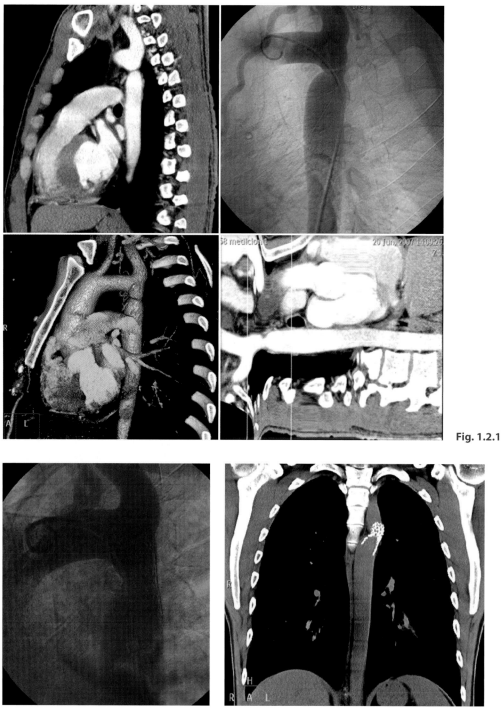

Fig. 1.2.1

Fig. 1.2.2   Fig. 1.2.3

A 35-year-old male with history of hypertension and subarachnoid hemorrhage (SAH) because of rupture of the anterior communicating artery aneurysm complained of chest pain and leg weakness. Physical examination revealed upper extremity hypertension and diminished femoral pulsations; telesistolic ejective murmur irradiated to interescapular region. ECG with left ventricle hypertrophy (LVH), MSCT was performed to evaluate the aorta anatomy.

Comments

Coarctation of the aorta (CoA) accounts for 5–10% of congenital heart disease and occurs frequently in whites and males. CoA usually consists of a narrowing of the aorta lumen that can take place at any level of its length, but most often occurs distally to the origin of the left subclavian artery near the insertion of the ligamentum arteriosum. This pathology should not be considered as a simple and isolated anomaly but as a diffuse arteriopathy with propensity to formation of aneurysms and dissections remote to the site of coarctation. In addition, more than 50% of patients have an associated BAV and 10% of patients have cerebral aneurysms, suggesting a common etiologic mechanism. The clinical manifestations depend on the location and degree of stenosis, the age, and the presence of cardiac abnormalities associated. Most patients develop persistent systemic hypertension, often as children, and are at risk for premature CAD. Other symptoms may be headaches, nosebleeds, cool extremities, leg weakness, or claudication with exertion. More serious manifestations include angina and heart failure. Cardiovascular examination may identify a systolic ejection murmur at the left upper sternal border that radiates to the interescapular area, upper extremity hypertension usually in conjunction with diminished and delayed femoral pulsations. The EKG could be normal or show left ventricular hypertrophy in older children and young adults. Potential complications include catastrophic aortic rupture or dissection and cerebral berry aneurysm rupture.

The mean survival for untreated patients is 38 years. In the long-term follow-up the leading cause of death is myocardial infarction; that is why in patients older than 30 years it is necessary to assess the existence of CAD. The most important predictor of survival is the age of treatment. MSCT is a very powerful method for making a diagnosis and for the follow-up of patients because of its capabilities for the aortic visualization and for coronary status assessment.

Imaging Findings

A noninvasive coronary and aortic angiotomography was performed. Functional analysis was performed for anatomical evaluation of aortic valve. Aortic valve evidenced bicuspids, aortic ring had a diameter of 27 mm, ascending aorta was 56 × 56 mm at the level of the pulmonary artery bifurcation.

Narrowing of the aorta lumen was seen below the left subclavian artery. The assessment of the aortic coarctation showed a proximal diameter of 16 mm, with 20 mm in the distal segment and a total length of 36 mm (Fig. 1.2.1).

In assessing coronary artery tree no significant CAD was evidenced.

These findings were correlated with invasive aortic and coronary angiography.

The patient underwent percutaneous angioplasty of the aorta with stent (Fig. 1.2.2).

MSCT follow-up was done 6 months later which showed correct placement and expansion of stent (Fig. 1.2.3).

Case 1.3

◼
Follow-Up of Coronary Aneurysm Post Pharmacological Stent Implantation

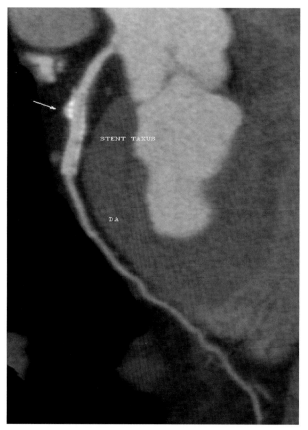

Fig. 1.3.1

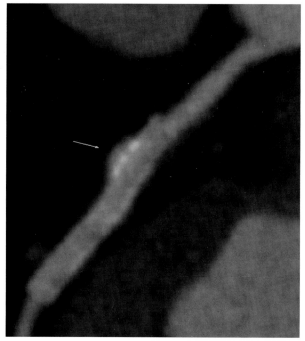

Fig. 1.3.2

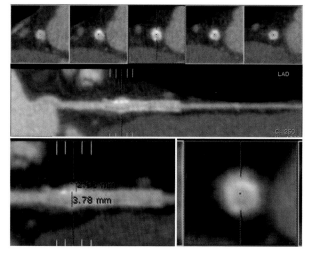

Fig. 1.3.3

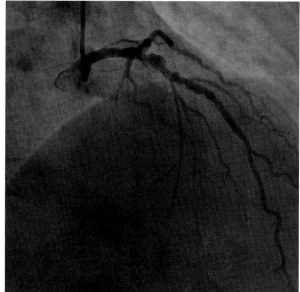

Fig. 1.3.4

A 50-year-old, male with smoking as coronary risk factor and history of coronary artery percutaneous angioplasty with drug-eluting stent (DES) placement (TAXUS paclitaxel-eluting stent (PES)) in LAD, was admitted to our clinic for invasive coronary angiography (ICA) due to a perfusion test that revealed inferior ischemia. The ICA showed a severe lesion in right coronary artery (RCA) and a patent stent in LAD with the finding of an aneurysmatic dilatation on the site of the implant of stent TAXUS. Six months later it was decided to perform an MSCT as follow-up of the LAD aneurysm.

Comments

Complications, such as acute and subacute thrombosis, inadequate late apposition phenomena, and coronary aneurysms (CA) at the implantation site, have been reported with DES. The incidence of coronary aneurysm after the use of drug-eluting stents is currently unknown and their clinical evolution is poorly understood.

In the treatment of de novo CAD using a single PES (Taxus V) trial the incidence was 1.4% with Taxus stent, compared with 0.2% prevalence with bare metal stent (p = 0.07).

In a case report, Bavry et al. described four patients with coronary aneurysm in both sirolimus and paclitaxel DES; two of these had concomitant bare metal stents (BMS), and coexisting aneurysm in these stents were not described.

The major prevalence of CA with DES compared with BMS led to speculation on possible hypersensitivity to the drug, although the pathophysiological mechanism causing the dilation has not been determined precisely. Evidence of inflammation related to the drug, polymer, or metal has been described, as well as persistent inflammatory phenomena, with a delay in endothelization of the stent area in tissues exposed to polymer or drug. Pathologic examination of the aneurysm revealed eosinophilic infiltration.

The lack of physiopathological and prognostic information, the unknown natural course of the condition, and the potential complications of CA hinder therapeutic decision. Long-term clinical follow-up of patients with DES, and in-depth clinical and experimental studies on possible chronic inflammatory processes are needed. MSCT provides an interesting noninvasive tool for diagnosis and follow-up of this rare complication.

Findings

A dynamic noninvasive coronary angiotomography was performed with a 64-row-detector scan after the intravenous administration of nonionic contrast. The coronary segmentation was established in 2D and 3D volume rendering. Coronary evaluation at curve multiplanar reconstruction showed a patent stent in mid-LAD correctly expanded in all its length (Fig. 1.3.1). In proximal LAD, an aneurismatic dilatation outside the metal structure in the superior border was suspected (Fig. 1.3.2). In the longitudinal analysis of the vessel, a diameter of 3.78 mm was observed between the superior and the inferior wall of the stent and a diameter of 2.12 mm between the upper wall of the stent and the upper wall of the vessel, which might be associated with the aneurismatic dilatation at that level (Fig. 1.3.3).

All these findings were correctly correlated with invasive coronary artery angiography (Fig. 1.3.4).

Case 1.4
■
Imaging Integration in Coronary Artery Disease

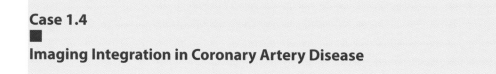

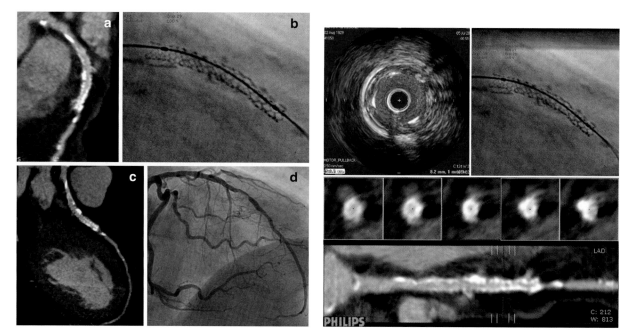

Fig. 1.4.1

Fig. 1.4.3

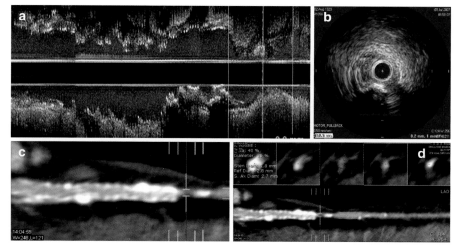

Fig. 1.4.2

A 72-year-old male, hypertensive and dislipidemic and with a history of percutaneous coronary angiography (PTCA) with two stents in LAD (one DES, one BMS), complained of atypical chest pain and presented a perfusion test with mild apical ischemia. Due to his past medical history, an MSCT was indicated to evaluate CAD. With the findings obtained in MSCT the patient underwent ICA and angioplasty, using rotational angiography, intravascular ultrasound (IVUS), and stent boost as complementary methods.

Comments

Atherosclerosis is a disease process that originates on the vessel walls of coronary arteries. ICA has traditionally served as the principal imaging modality to evaluate CAD; however, this method shows only the lumen artery but not the wall. IVUS is an invasive diagnostic method that evaluates the lumen and the vessel wall. It allows not only the quantification of CAD but also its characterization, as for example soft plaque, calcified plaque, etc. Since 1998, MSCT has been used as a diagnostic method that can also evaluate wall and lumen vessel but in a noninvasive way. Due to the fact that both methods evaluate lumen and wall artery vessel, IVUS is taken as the gold standard for that assessment in comparatives studies with MSCT. Multiples studies have been performed for correlation between ICA and MSCT for the assessment of grades of coronary stenosis. Actually ICA has improved diagnostic accuracy for CAD with new technology as rotational angiography that allows evaluating the vessel in different projections with only one injection of contrast, decreasing the contrast volume required and the radiation exposure. Another technique named "Stent Boost" (performed during the angioplasty) allows the subtraction of the image of the stent implanted for the evaluation of the correct expansion of it. In conclusion, in this presented case MSCT allowed the diagnostic evaluation of CAD and to choose the better therapeutic strategy of percutaneous revascularization.

Findings

Figure 1.4.1 (a–c) MSCT curve multiplanar reconstruction showing a stent in proximal LAD and a severe lesion at the distal edge of the stent. Findings correlated with stent boost (b) and ICA (d).

Figure 1.4.2 (a, b) IVUS images (bidimensional and longitudinal views) that show a severe lesion at the end of the stent in mid-LAD associated with a mix plaque (calcified in hour 6 and soft plaque from hour 7 to 1) placed in an artery of 3 × 2.75 mm. Correlation with vessel analysis by MSCT (c, d).

Figure 1.4.3 IVUS images showing the infraexpansion of the stent with concentric soft plaque behind the struts of the stent. Correlation with vessel analysis of MSCT and with stent boost.

Case 1.5
■
Cath Laboratory Planning

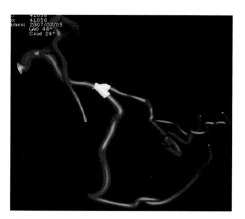

Fig. 1.5.1

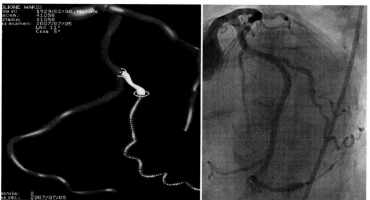

Fig. 1.5.2

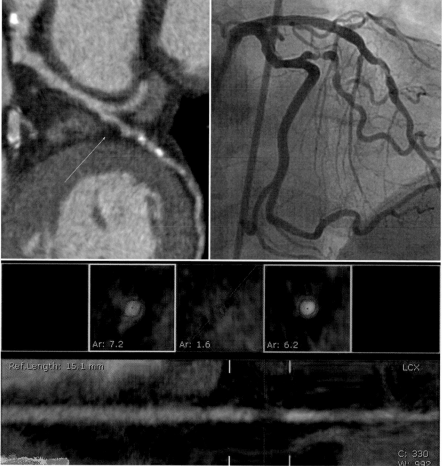

Fig. 1.5.3

A 70-year-old male has a complete left bundle block with a 5-year history of coronary angioplasty to LAD with stent (the rest of the coronary arteries were without significant lesion). Because of an equivocal stress test a coronary MSCT was perfomed. On discovering a severe lesion at bifurcation of the circumflex artery (CX), percutaneous revascularization of the obstructing lesion was planned using a technique named "coronary angiography with three-dimensional tomography reconstruction" (True View®) as postprocessing.

Coronary angiography with three-dimensional tomography reconstruction (True View®) is a 64-detector multislice tomograph tool that allows us to display the coronary arteries in all views emphasizing the assessment of bifurcation lesions and ostial lesions, allowing in this way to predict prior to an invasive procedure (PTCA) the best angiographic view to evaluate the segment of interest and its treatment.

This tool allows us to measure with high accuracy the diameter and the length of the segment to evaluate and/or treat, and also allows the choice of the best endoprosthesis (stent) to get the right diameter and length and optimize the therapeutic outcome, finally defining the best view to plan a procedure that ensures minimum radiation to the patient and the operators, and that also uses minimum contrast material preserving all its benefits.

The true view images can be transferred from the tomography work station to the cath laboratory where the invasive procedure is to take place.

Figure 1.5.1 Tridimensional reconstruction of left coronary artery showing in right caudal oblique projection a bifurcation lesion that compromises the ostium and the proximal segment of obtuse marginal branch (OM) of CX. It shows the diameter and length of bifurcation of CX and OM.

Figure 1.5.2 Utility of 3D reconstruction for the quantification and evaluation of the length of the ostial and proximal lesion in OM. Image correlated with ICA.

Figure 1.5.3 MSCT: vessel analysis (bottom) with measurement of utility for lab cath planning and curve multiplanar reconstruction (top) (correlated with ICA) where it shows a bifurcation lesion in mid-CX that compromises the ostial and proximal segment of OM branch (associated with soft plaque in the proximal segment and mid-segment calcified plaque) (arrow).

Case 1.6

■

MSCT and Left Main Coronary Artery Stenting Evaluation

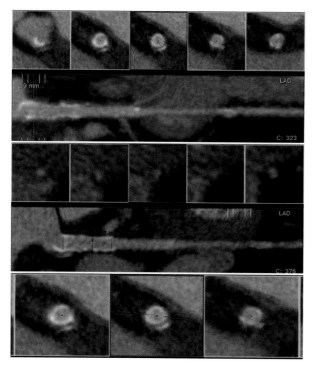

Fig. 1.6.1

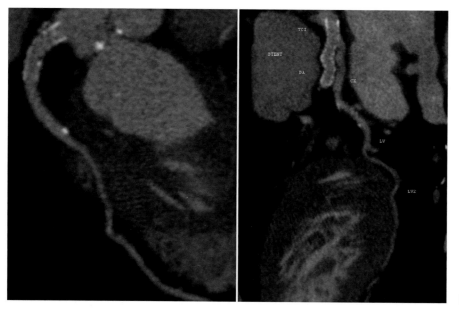

Fig. 1.6.2

A 65-year-old female patient, with smoking and high cholesterol as coronary risk factors, has a history of stable angina NHYA III–IV and PTCA with stent placement at proximal left main coronary artery (LM). She presents 4 months later with atypical chest pain and an equivocal stress test. MSCT was performed to evaluate the patency of the stent.

Comments

Surgery is still the recommended treatment for significant left main (LM) disease although the introduction of drug-eluting stents (DES) with much lower restenosis rates has increasingly resulted in the alternative use of percutaneous coronary intervention (PCI).

The expert consensus suggests ICA 6 months after PCI to left main coronary intervention due to the unpredictable occurrence of in-stent restenosis (ISR) and in relation with sudden cardiac death. Current MSCT technology, in combination with optimal heart rate control, allows accurate evaluation of selected patients after LM angioplasty. Neointimal hyperplasia within the stent can be visualized demonstrating its potential for the detection of ISR, in addition to stent patency. It is important to use appropriate window and threshold levels to obtain adequate images.

Vam Mieghem et al., in a recent study published in Circulation, evaluated the diagnostic accuracy of MSCT to detect ISR after stenting of the LM. MSCT correctly identified all patients with ISR (10 of 70). The accuracy of MSCT for detection of angiographic ISR was 98% for the evaluation of patients with stenting of the LM and for those with distal LM bifurcation lesions, in whom only one of the major branch vessels is stented. In complex bifurcation the accuracy was less (83%). For the assessment of stent diameter and area, MSCT showed good correlation with intravascular ultrasound.

A negative MSCT can rule out the presence of LM ISR and may be an acceptable first-line alternative to ICA in a subset of patients.

Imaging Findings

Coronaries evaluation showed, at the level of the LM coronary artery, a stent in direction to the LAD. The stent had a width of 20 mm, with a diameter of 4.9 mm in the proximal segment, 4.47 mm in the middle segment, and 4.47 mm in the distal segment (vessel analysis reconstruction, see Fig. 1.6.1). A patent stent was demonstrated. The LAD was a long artery of moderate caliber. It gave origin to average caliber diagonals and septal perforator branches. There were moderate amounts of nonobstructing soft plaques in the mid-LAD. There was no disease in the distal LAD. The left circumflex (Cx) was a moderate caliber artery of average length. It gave origin to two obtuse marginal branches. There were diffuse soft plaques with a mild to moderate ostial obstruction (curve multiplanar reconstruction of LM LAD and Cx, see Fig. 1.6.2). The RCA was a moderate caliber artery with no significant disease. With information of the patency of the stent assessed with this method the patient did not need any further invasive studies.

Case 1.7
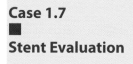
Stent Evaluation

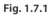

Fig. 1.7.1

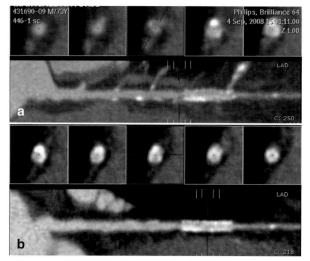

Fig. 1.7.2

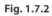

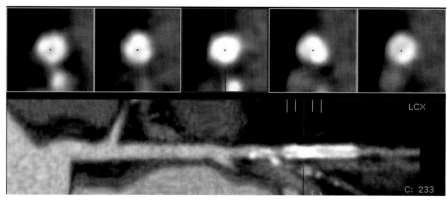

Fig. 1.7.3

A 64-year-old male, with hypercholesterolemia and hypertension as coronary risk factors who had previously undergone percutaneous transluminal coronary angioplasty in combination with stent placement was readmitted to our hospital with recurrent angina. MSCT was performed prior to conventional coronary angiography in order to assess stent patency noninvasively.

Comments

In comparison to ICA, 16- or 64-slice CT has been shown to permit the detection of coronary artery stenoses in native coronary arteries with a high sensitivity and specificity of up to 99% and 98%, respectively.

The clinical incidence of restenosis after coronary stent implantation is 20–35% for BMS and 5–10% for drug-eluting stents (DES). Recently, MSCT has emerged as a potential non-invasive imaging method in the evaluation of stents. The rate of evaluable stents by CT is low. Even in assessable stents, several factors that influence the evaluation of stent patency by CT have been identified, such as stent diameter, type of stent, site of stent implantation, high calcium load, motion artifacts, and contrast resolution.

Stent-related high-density artifacts lead to artificial narrowing of the lumen, leaving only a small portion of the in-stent lumen visible, thus making reliable detection of subtle hyperplasia extremely difficult. The size of stent is an important factor that impairs evaluation of stent patency by CT. Those with a diameter <3 mm cannot be correctly evaluated. Rixe et al. reported that 58% of stents, which had a mean diameter of 3.28 mm, were evaluable by 64-slice CT, and that the mean diameter of invaluable stents was 3.03 mm. The metallic part (thickness of strut) of DES might also be a factor that impairs evaluation of stent patency. The metallic part of DES tends to be thicker than that of BMS, and the diameter of DES (2.5–3.5 mm) tends to be smaller than that of BMS; however, type of stent (DES or BMS) is not a significant predictor for agreement of findings between CT and ICA.

There are some subject-related factors that also impair evaluation of stent patency such as high heart rate (HR), presence of arrhythmia, high body weight and body mass index (BMI), and high calcium load.

In evaluable stents, MSCT has a high negative predictive value and moderate positive predictive value to exclude ISR.

Imaging Findings

Figure 1.7.1 LAD Curve multiplanar reconstruction: showing stent-like image in mid-segment that looks patent and magnified image with severe lumen narrowing at the proximal edge of stent (arrow) image compatible with ISR.

Figure 1.7.2 LAD longitudinal vessel analysis and cross-sectional of the ISR at the proximal edge of the stent (a) and stent patency (b).

Figure 1.7.3 LCX longitudinal vessel analysis and cross-sectional showing artifact due to metallic struts of the stent that make the correct assessment of its patency difficult.

Case 1.8
■
Coronary Anomalies

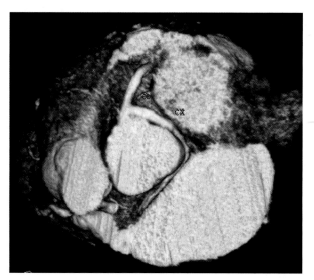

Fig. 1.8.1

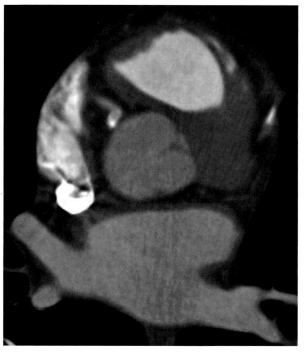

Fig. 1.8.2

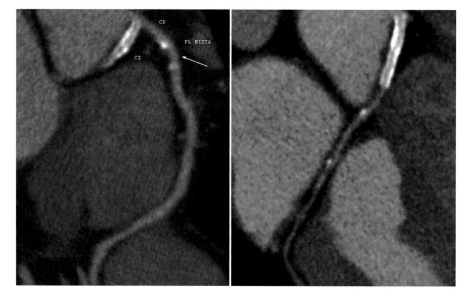

Fig. 1.8.3

A 42-year-old male, hypertensive with a 3-year history of PTCA with stent implantation at left circumflex artery (LCX) complained of chest pain with a perfusion test nondiagnostic for ischemia. MSCT was done to evaluate CAD and patency of the stent.

Comments

Coronary artery anomalies may be part of complex congenital malformation of the heart such as transposition, tetralogy, or truncus arteriosus or may be an isolated defect.

They are relatively uncommon, occurring in 0.2–1.2% of the population. They were thought to be insignificant, but are well known to be the cause of sudden death.

Normally the RCA takes origin perpendicular from the right anterior sinus of Valsalva and the LAD and LCX from the left sinus. There are different types of coronary origin anomalies: LAD from pulmonary trunk, LAD from right aortic sinus, LAD from posterior aortic sinus, RCA artery from left aortic sinus, LCX from the right aortic sinus or from the RCA itself, i.e., high takeoff of RCA.

Clinical manifestations can be angina, myocardial infarction, syncope and ventricular arrhythmias, and sudden death, frequently precipitated by effort. Sudden death is related to myocardial ischemia, several potential mechanism have been postulated to explain it. First, because of the acute takeoff the ostium of the anomalous coronary is slit-like and, second, the first segment of the vessel runs between the aorta and the pulmonary trunk making it susceptible to compression due to expansion of these arteries.

Origin of LCX from very proximal RCA or from right aortic sinus is considered the most frequent congenital coronary artery anomaly. The anomalous artery may arise as a proximal branch of the RCA from the same ostium of the RCA or from a separate orifice in the right aortic sinus. The anomalous vessel shows an initial retroartic course between the aorta and the atrial wall merging in the atrioventricular sulcus to pursue its usual final distribution.

Therefore, unlike other aberrant coronary arteries passing between the aorta and pulmonary trunk, there is no apparent risk of extrinsic compression and this anomaly is considered meaningless with regard to myocardial ischemia.

However, there are descriptions of sudden death and myocardial infarction in these patients with neither evidence of atherosclerotic CAD nor angiographic evidence of compression of the vessel at its retroaortic course. Some authors consider this anomaly as a predisposing cause of accelerated developing of atherosclerotic plaque and there are descriptions of major prevalence of CAD at the proximal course of the anomaly coronary.

Findings

Figure 1.8.1 and 1.8.2 MSCT: 3D volume rendering (Fig 1.8.1) and axial images (Fig 1.8.2) show the coronary origin anomaly of LCX from the RCA. There is a patent stent in proximal segment of LCX. RCA is a large vessel of important caliber with a mix plaque (soft and calcified), no flow limiting, in the proximal segment.

Figure 1.8.3 Curve multiplanar reconstructing of RCA and LCX.

Case 1.9
■
Stent Fracture

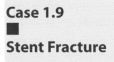

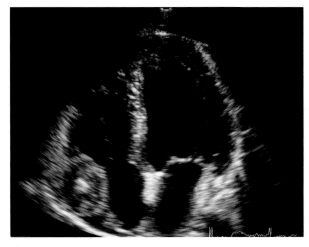

Fig. 1.9.1   Fig. 1.9.2

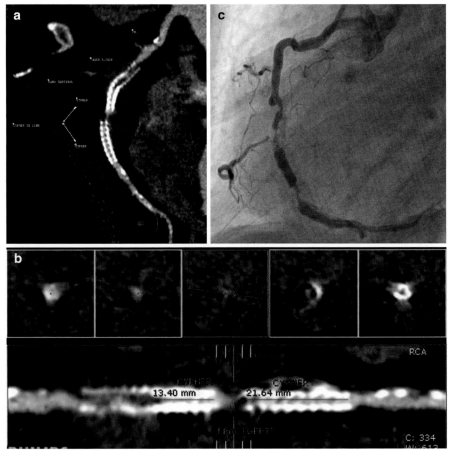

Fig. 1.9.3

A 47-year-old male with family history of hypercholesterolemia has a 15-year history of coronary angioplasty with bare metal stent in mid RCA. During the past year he had progressive angina with evidence of ISR, so a second stent ((PES) Taxus) was placed intra-stent. Six months later, angina and inducible ischemia reappeared; ICA showed ISR of the second stent, so a third overlapping stent (33 × 3 mm sirolimus-eluting stent, (SES) Cypher) was placed. Lately, he had recurrent angina with inferior ischemia in stress echo and a mass in the right atrioventricular groove that motivates the performance of a MSCT and ICA.

Comments

Several complications have been described with drug-eluting stents (DES) such as acute thrombosis, ISR, aneurisms, and fracture.

The incidence of stent fracture is low (1.7–7.7%) in different studies. The clinical mani-festation could be: stable and unstable angina, ST elevation myocardial infarction, and potentially sudden death. Factors that increase the risk of fracture are lengthy stents, high inflation pressure, right coronary stent location, vein graft stent, and overlapping stents. This complication was described predominantly with SES rather than PES stents.

Several mechanisms have been proposed to explain this complication such as metal fatigue caused by repetitive compressions, kinking and shear stresses in stents placed in tortuous angled vessels, increased wall motion along the RCA, axial rigidity of the overlap-ping stent segments, and higher radial forces in lengthy stents.

The increased rate of fracture in SES over PES (Taxus®, Boston Scientific, Natick, Massachusetts, USA) might be related to the closed-cell design of the former compared to the open design of the PES. The closed-cell design does offer some benefit including more regular strut distribution allowing more predictable local drug delivery and lower intimal growth rates. Complications of coronary artery stent fractures include restenosis and thrombosis at the site of fracture.

In this case the patient had several predictors of stent fracture, lengthy stents, SES, implantation at RCA, and overlapping stents. All these factors were correctly assessed by MSCT.

Findings

Figure 1.9.1 Echo 2D Imaging: cystic-appearing mass of 3 × 3 mm, surrounding a very echogenic structure, seemingly metallic, in contact with the right AV groove adjacent to the location of the stents.

Figure 1.9.2 MSCT axial image which correlates with the echo findings.

Figure 1.9.3 (a–c) Curve multiplanar reconstruction and longitudinal vessel analysis (LVA) images showing the RCA with stent taxus overlapped with SES 33 × 3 mm which has a continuity solution and ISR in taxus stent. Images correlated with ICA.

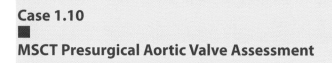

Case 1.10

MSCT Presurgical Aortic Valve Assessment

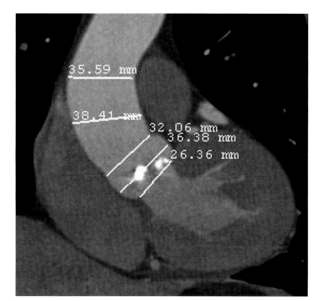

Fig. 1.10.1

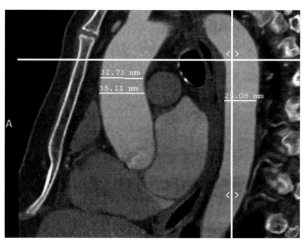

Fig. 1.10.2

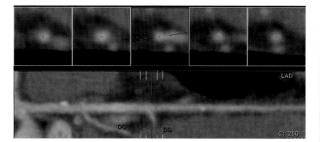

Fig. 1.10.3

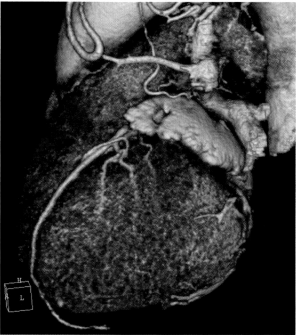

Fig. 1.10.4

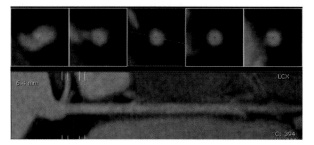

Fig. 1.10.5

A 65-year-old male with severe progression of an aortic stenosis was selected for valve replacement surgery. He was an athlete with good functional ability, with an dyslipidemia controlled with medication, no history of CAD. A MSCT was programmed to access coronary anatomy before surgery.

Comments

Guidelines of cardiologist societies recommend routine invasive coronary evaluation for most patients who need to undergo valve heart surgery for repair or replacement. The presence of concomitant obstructive CAD in patients undergoing cardiac valvular surgery worsens prognosis. Various studies have shown that combined valve and bypass surgery of significant CAD reduced early and late mortality. Because aortic stenosis and CAD share common risk factors, concomitant significant CAD is not an uncommon finding in these patients.

Abnormal stress studies, such as echo and nuclear tests, lack of sufficient accuracy for reliable detection of concomitant CAD. The diagnostic performance of 64-slice CT scanners to detect coronary stenoses is very good in patients who have a high prevalence of CAD. In these patients the negative predictive value of 64-slice CT scanners is very high, allowing the exclusion of the presence of significant CAD. MSCT can assess morphological parameters in addition to the coronary evaluation, such as aortic annulus, sinotubular junction, and ascending and descending aorta dimensions that can be very useful to the surgeon to choose the technical approach. Also useful is the measurement of left ventricular cavities' diameters and function with the possibility to assess end diastolic volume, end systolic volume, and ejection fraction, which are major outcomes predictors in this set of patients. It is possible that in the near future, a combination of noninvasive coronary angiography with MSCT and echocardiography will be enough to decide the performance of valvular surgery.

Imaging Findings

This patient showed no aortic dilatation, left atrium enlargement, normal left ventricular dimension and three leaflet aortic valve. Left ventricular diastolic diameter was 51 mm, systolic 28 mm, septum 10 mm, left atrium 47 mm. Ascending aorta was 41–42 mm and descending aorta 25–24 mm (at the pulmonary artery bifurcation) (Figs. 1.10.1–1.10.2).

Left main coronary artery was of important length and large caliber, trifurcating into the LAD, ramus, and left circumflex coronary artery. The LAD was a long artery of important caliber giving origin to three average-caliber diagonal branches. There were moderate amounts of fibrocalcified plaques in the proximal and mid-LAD, without flow-limiting stenosis. There was no disease in the distal LAD (Fig. 1.10.3 shows vessel analysis; Fig. 1.10.4 shows 3D volume rendering of LAD). Left circumflex coronary artery was dominant, giving origin to obtuse marginal branches with no significant lesions (Fig. 1.10.5). The RCA was a short artery of moderate caliber with no significant CAD.

With these results the patient was sent to surgery with no extra coronary evaluation.

Case 1.11
■
MSCT Coronary Assessment Prior to Mitral Valve Surgery

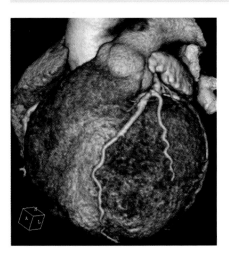

Fig. 1.11.1

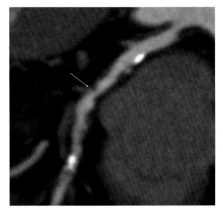

Fig. 1.11.2

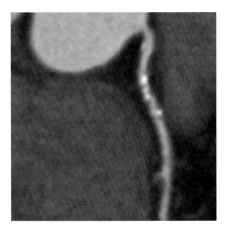

Fig. 1.11.6

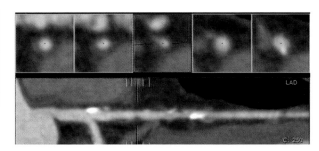

Fig. 1.11.3

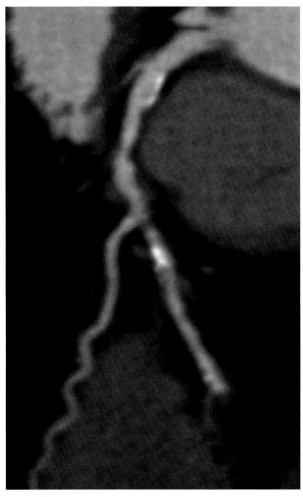

Fig. 1.11.4

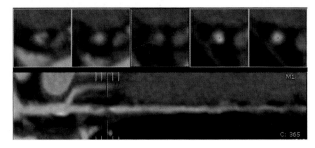

Fig. 1.11.5

A 70-year-old male with hypertension and smoking as coronary risk factors and no history of CAD, had severe mitral valve insufficiency due to rupture of chordae tendineae diagnosed by echocardiography with no other findings. It was assumed to be idiopathic. The left ventricular function was normal. He had no symptoms at all. His referral physician sent him to perform an MSCT to rule out CAD, trying to better define the needs of surgery.

Comments

Patients who are scheduled to undergo open heart surgery with purely regurgitant valves, often do not need concomitant CABG but mitral regurgitation could be the consequence of CAD, as significant CAD is found in approximately one-third of these patients.

The American College of Cardiology/AHA committee indicates preoperative coronary angiography in symptomatic patients and/or those with left ventricular dysfunction in men >35 years, premenopausal women >35 years with risk factors for CAD, and postmenopausal women. Noninvasive coronary angiography with MSCT appears to be an interesting method to assess CAD in this set of patients. With the latest 64-slice CT scanners the accuracy to detect coronary stenoses is very good in patients who have a high prevalence of CAD. In these patients the negative predictive value is very high, allowing to exclude the presence of significant CAD. Knowing that the sensitivity and specificity to detect severe CAD is not 100%, it is still necessary to perform coronary angiography to confirm the results of MSCT. Recent development in MSCT permits the postprocessing of the mitral valve being possible in order to have an anatomic visualization of the valve, including also functional information after reconstructing all phases of the cardiac cycle. This information serves as a complement to the echo helping the surgeon to define the better therapeutic strategy. The aorta and cavities dimensions are also assessed. The MSCT angiography technology will probably advance to avoid any presurgical invasive test in case of mitrol valve replacement.

Findings

Multiplanar reconstruction, 3D volume rendering, and LVA of left main (LM) and anterior descending artery (LAD) showed LM of important length and large caliber. There was a mild calcified nonobstructing plaque. The LAD was a long artery of large caliber. There was a soft plaque in the proximal LAD, with moderate to severe stenosis. There was no disease in the distal LAD (Figs. 1.11.1–1.11.3). The first diagonal had a moderate soft plaque (Fig. 1.11.4). The left circumflex was dominant; it had large caliber and important length. It gave origin to an important obtuse marginal (OM1) branch that had a proximal severe stenosis associated with a soft plaque: LVA of OM1 (Fig. 1.11.5). The RCA was an artery of moderate caliber. There was a moderate ostial obstruction due to a soft plaque and nonobstructing calcified plaques in the proximal segment (Fig. 1.11.6). Our suggestion was to correlate these findings with a coronary invasive angiography due to the possibility of a combined surgery.

Case 1.12
■
Coronary Total Occlusion: Preintervention Assessment

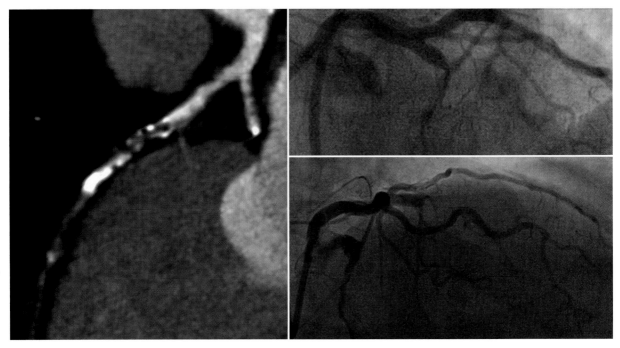

Fig. 1.12.1

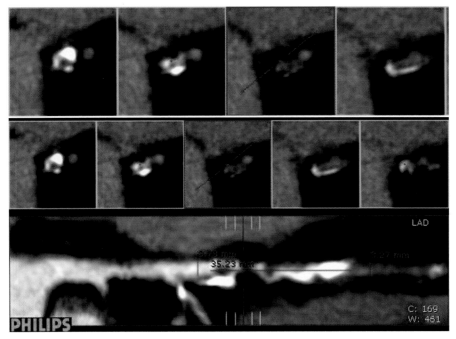

Fig. 1.12.2

A 70-year-old male, who presented dyslipidemia, hypertension and type II diabetes mellitus, had a history of chronic stable angina and EKG with anterior myocardial infarction sequel.

A perfusion test demonstrated necrosis and perinecrosis ischemia in anterior territory.

ICA evidenced LAD coronary total occlusion (CTO), with no other obstructing lesions. MSCT was requested for CTO evaluation prior to revascularization treatment.

Comments

Preprocedural coronary lesion assessment by MSCT could offer strategic guidance in the setting of elective complex percutaneous coronary intervention (PCI). CT images of the target lesion served as a preprocedural road map depicting the bends of complex luminal path, vessel geometry, and occluded segment of the vessel. In the presence of CTO, coronary artery may not be visualized by selective coronary angiography while MSCT simultaneously could show the distal vessel filling from collateral vessels from the homo or contralateral artery. This method has the advantage of allowing the assessment of the occlusion length, qualitative characteristics of the occlusive plaque (type of plaque: soft, calcified), characteristics of the lumen, and anatomy of the vessel distal to the occlusive lesion, and measurement of diameters proximal and distal to the occlusive lesion.

Assessment of the occlusion length and the presence of calcium in the occluding atherosclerotic plaque have been found to be independent predictors of procedural outcome. Occlusion length >15 mm and the presence of severe calcification have been found to be independent predictors of procedural failure.

With all this information the interventional cardiologist could infer the chances of crossing the lesion, achieving the optimal strategy and material for treating a CTO and the posterior revascularization of it, with the best guiding catheter, wire, balloon, and stent in relation to the type of CTO.

In conclusion, MSCT is a very important method that acurately assesses the CTO and allows the interventional cardiologist to perform, or not, the revascularization in order to achieve the best result and the lowest restenosis at long-term follow-up.

Imaging Findings

Figure 1.12.1 Curve multiplanar reconstructing (MPRc) of LAD: diffuse disease with severe calcification in mid-segment where a total occlusion (CTO) is seen. After the CTO, there are soft plaques with moderate obstruction of the lumen in a thin vessel. Image correlated with ICA.

Figure 1.12.2 Longitudinal vessel analysis of LAD and cross-sectional images showing a large soft and calcified plaque with a complete stop marked with an oblique line in the cross-sectional images. This series also includes the assessment of vessel diameter at the beginning and at the end of the lesion and the total length of it.

Case 1.13
■
Utility of MSCT in Acute Coronary Syndrome

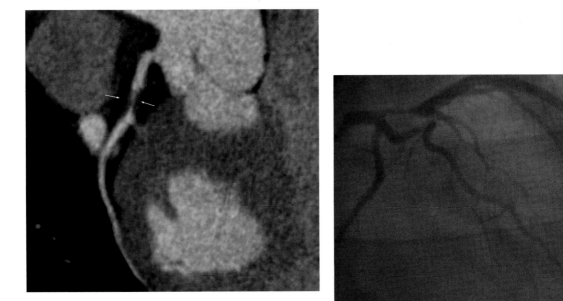

Fig. 1.13.1

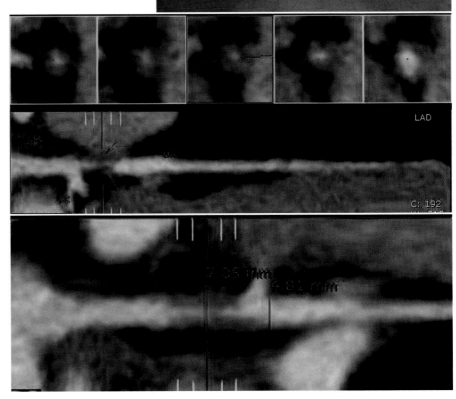

Fig. 1.13.2

A 45-year-old male, smoker with a history of hypertension complained of atypical chest pain and dysnea; the electrocardiogram showed giant T waves with no ST changes.

He was admitted to rule out acute coronary syndrome (ACS) in our chest pain unit protocol. An MSCT was performed for triple rule out.

Comments

Chest pain is a frequent chief complaint in the Emergency Department. Given the suspicion of chest pain of coronary etiology the usual screening is to perform serial EKG, measure markers in blood, and finally, as appropriate, conduct a functional test. One of the challenges in important cardiovascular centers is to be able to rule out in patients with chest pain for their higher morbidity the three more risky causes: acute aortic syndrome (AAS), pulmonary embolism, and ACS. MSCT can evaluate these three entities.

The advantage of performing MSCT in this group of patients is its high diagnostic certainty to exclude the presence of coronary disease because of its high negative predictive value. In presence of CAD, it quantifies the degree of coronary stenosis, and analyzes within the coronary obstructions what could correspond to the culprit plaque observed on clinical examination.

As it has been demonstrated by IVUS, characteristics that predict the instability of the plaque responsible for the ACS are: the presence of soft plaque, positive remodeling, and eccentricity. MSCT as a noninvasive alternative can assess the overall measurement of all existing plaques, and evaluate their severity and characteristics.

The ultimate goal is to determine not only the severity but also the culprit lesion responsible for the patient's symptom.

There are three findings that are related to the instability of the plaque (responsible plaque): soft plaque (noncalcified plaque with a density <30 HU), plaque with spotty calcification (mix plaque with calcified lesions <3 mm), and positive remodeling (remodeling index on MSCT is calculated as positive remodeling when the diameter at the plaque site is at least 10% larger than the reference segment).

A study that assessed the characteristics of the culprit lesion by MSCT in patients with ACS before ICA, found that the presence of all these three factors showed a high positive predictive value, and the absence of all three showed a high negative predictive value for the identification of the culprit plaques.

It is logical to presume that plaques vulnerable to rupture harbor similar characteristics.

The case presented evidenced the presence of soft plaque and positive remodeling, with severe obstruction of the lumen. MSCT not only allowed diagnosing but also determining the therapeutic option (percutaneous revascularization).

Imaging Findings

Figure 1.13.1 Curve multiplanar reconstruction (MPRc): ostial and proximal severe obstruction of LAD because of concentric lesion associated with soft plaque and positive remodeling. ICA correlated image.

Figure 1.13.2 Longitudinal vessel analysis: assessment of proximal and distal diameter of the lesion and its length. Hounsfield units determination of soft plaque and positive remodeling.

Case 1.14
■
Accuracy of MSCT for Assessment of Coronary Artery Disease

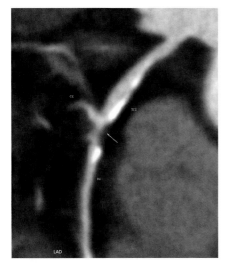

Fig. 1.14.1

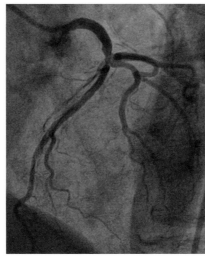

Fig. 1.14.2

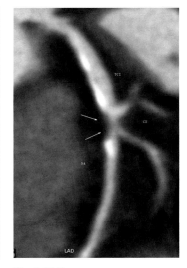

Fig. 1.14.3

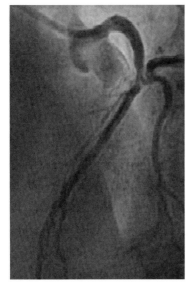

Fig. 1.14.4

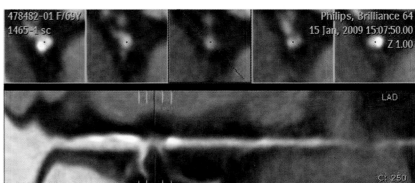

Fig. 1.14.5

A 62-year-old female, with hypertension and dislipidemia as coronary risk factors and no history of CAD, complained of atypical chest pain and had an abnormal stress test. She was asked to undergo an MSCT to rule out CAD.

Multidetector CT scanners with faster imaging speed allow high spatial resolution and sufficient temporal resolution to permit adequate and reliable visualization of the coronary artery lumen. Faster rotation times and lower heart rates positively influence the diagnostic accuracy.

Comparison to ICA demonstrates increasing accuracy for stenosis detection. Severe coronary calcifications remain a problem because they can impair image quality and reduce diagnostic accuracy. The published studies uniformly reported high sensitivities for the detection of coronary artery stenosis, ranging from 82 to 95%. Similarly, specificity for stenosis detection ranged from 86 to 98%. Of note, the negative predictive value was uniformly found to be 97% or higher, but it has to be considered that the low prevalence of significant coronary stenoses influences the negative predictive value toward higher levels. Clinical application in patients with a high pretest likelihood for CAD is of limited value; if the predicted necessity for an intervention is reasonably high, the patient should proceed directly to invasive angiography rather than CT. Also, routine "screening" of asymptomatic individuals by CCTA will not be beneficial, since treatment of an asymptomatic stenosis is controversial. Patients symptomatic with atypical chest pain and positive or equivocal stress test results, with low or intermediate pretest likelihood are candidates for noninvasive coronary angiography.

CCTA has the unique ability to evaluate the wall of the artery as well as the coronary lumen. It is well known that patients with minimal CAD may still have events due to plaques which are not fully defined by ICA. These types of nonstenotic plaques are detectable by coronary CTA allowing the possibility of early medical intervention.

Coronary CTA remains a valuable tool in evaluating patients, for the presence of coronary disease and in making the determination as to whether or not further invasive testing is needed.

Curve multiplanar reconstruction of a CCTA (Figs. 1.14.1–1.14.3) and LVA (Fig. 1.14.5) showed a nonobstructing calcified eccentric lesion of the left main coronary artery, and an eccentric, moderate to severe lesion at the distal left main and ostium of LAD that is opposed to the origin of circumflex artery and ramus intermedius.

The MSCT allowed evaluating the characteristics of the lesion in view of the treatment of percutaneous revascularization determining the degree of obstruction, the length of the lesion, the best angiographic projection, and commitment from other vessels.

Correlation with invasive angiography prior to the PTCA performed on the patient (Figs. 1.14.2–1.14.4).

Case 1.15
■
MSCT Post-Coronary Bypass Surgery Evaluation

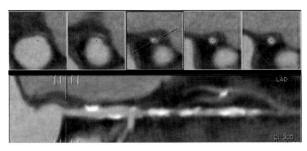

Fig. 1.15.1

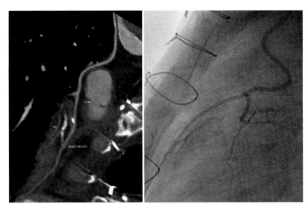

Fig. 1.15.2

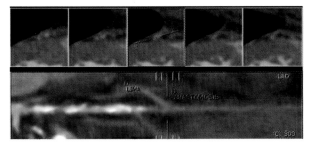

Fig. 1.15.3

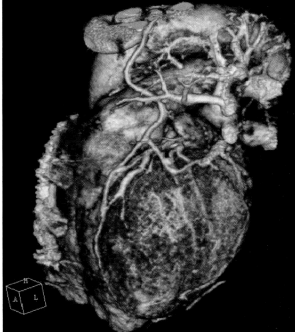

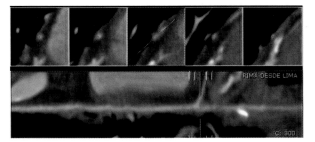

Fig. 1.15.4

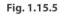

Fig. 1.15.5

A 60-year-old male, hypertensive, dislipidemic, smoker, and with family history of heart disease, presented with history of CABG: Left internal mammary artery (LIMA) to LAD, right internal mammary artery (RIMA) to circumflex (CX) and sequential to posterior descending artery of RCA (from LIMA). Because of worsening of his aerobic function capacity and findings from functional studies that generated suspicion of an ischemic area in the inferior territory he was referred to perform an MSCT scan to evaluate bypass status.

Comments

Because of latest success of CABG with improved long-term results, it is no longer current practice to perform routine invasive follow-up examination after revascularization. Only patients with evidence of recurrent ischemia or symptoms, undergo coronary angiography. A noninvasive method for obtaining reliable information on coronary artery anatomy would be of great value. The latest scanners appear to provide reliable detection of venous graft occlusion. Recent published reports and preliminary studies have observed that their accuracy in diagnosing venous graft occlusion is comparable to that of selective coronary angiography. Although it is more difficult to obtain good images of the smaller-diameter arterial grafts, compared with venous grafts, recent studies have reported 100% visibility. Accordingly, diagnosis of graft occlusion appears to be feasible. There are not enough data available on the ability to identify stenoses. Whereas the bypass body appears readily assessable, the region of the distal anastomosis (insertion site) remains problematic.

It is important to perform the study with attention to bypass grafts so that more of the ascending aorta is visualized.

Coronary CTA can be helpful, not only by delineating which grafts are patent, but by providing a "roadmap" of the number of grafts, their origins, as well as the placement of the anastomoses. It is important to evaluate not only the status of the patient's bypass grafts, but also that of the native coronary arteries. Evaluating post-bypass status is one of the most common indications to perform a noninvasive CTA.

Findings

There was severe disease and flow-limiting obstruction in the LM. There was severe diffuse disease in the proximal, mid-, and distal LAD. (MSCT-LVA) (Fig. 1.15.1). There was a patent arterial graft to mid-LAD with good opacification of the distal LAD. There was nonsignificant disease or stenosis in the body of the graft and the distal anastomosis (multiplanar curve reconstructing and ICA correlation Fig. 1.15.2 and LVA Fig. 1.15.3). There was severe obstructing plaque in the proximal obtuse marginal (OM) of the CX. The RCA was a long artery of great caliber. There were severe ostial and proximal lesion. Patent bypass RIMA (from the LIMA) to OM was with no significant disease (Fig. 1.15.4 LVA). The sequential graft from the OM to PDA was occluded. Figure 1.15.5 shows the 3D volume render image of the LIMA and RIMA. Conventional angiography confirmed the patency of LIMA and RIMA to OM and the occlusion of RIMA sequential to RCA continuing the procedure with angioplasty to RCA.

Further Reading

Books

Atlas of Non-Invasive Coronary Angiography by Multidetector Computed Tomography. Guillem Pons-Lladó, Rubén Leta-Petracca (eds) (2006) Springer, New York

Cardiac CT Imaging: Diagnosis of Cardiovascular Disease. Matthew J. Budoff, Jerold S. Shinbane (eds) (2006) Springer, New York

MRI and CT of the Cardiovascular System. Higgins CB, De Roos A (2005) Lippincott Williams & Wilkins, Philadelphia

Novel Techniques for Imaging the Heart. Marcelo F. Di Carli, Raymond Y. Kwong (eds) (2008) Wiley-Blackwell, Hoboken, NJ

MSCT Links

www.nasci.org (North American Society for Cardiac Imaging)

www.SCCT.org (Society of Cardiovascular Computed Tomography)

http://search.medscape.com/all-search

http://www.diagnosticimaging.com/imaging-trends-advances/cardiovascular-imaging

http://www.cardiosource.com/clinicalcollections/clinicalcollections.asp?CCID = 20

htpp://theonlinelearningcenter.com

Articles

Achenbach S, Giesler T, Ropers D, Ulzheimer S, Derlien H, Schulte C, Wenkel E, Moshage W, Bautz W, Daniel WG, Kalender WA, Baum U. Detection of coronary artery stenoses by contrast-enhanced, retrospectively electrocardiographically-gated, multislice spiral computed tomography. Circulation 2001; 103: 2535–2538

Achenbach S, Moselewski F, Ropers D et al Detection of calcified and noncalcified coronary atherosclerotic plaque by contrast-enhanced, submillimeter multidetector spiral computed tomography. Circulation 2004; 109:14–17

Achenbach S, Moshage W, Ropers D et al Value of EBCT for the noninvasive detection of high-grade coronary artery stenoses and occlusions. N Engl J Med 1998; 339:1964–1971

Achenbach S, Ropers D, Pohle FK, Raaz D, von Erffa J, Yilmaz A, Muschiol G, Daniel WG. Detection of coronary artery stenoses using multi-detector CT with 16 × 0.75 collimation and 375 ms rotation. Eur Heart J 2005; 26:1978–1986

Anders K et al Coronary bypass graft patency: assessment with high-resolution submillimeter 16-slice multidetector-row computed tomography versus coronary angiography. Eur J Radiol 2006; 57:336–344

Bashore TM, Bates ER, Berger PB et al; American College of Cardiology/Society for Cardiac Angiography and Interventions. Clinical expert consensus document on cardiac catheterization laboratory standards: a report of the American College of Cardiology Task Force on clinical expert consensus documents. J Am Coll Cardiol 2001; 37:2170–2214

Bashore TM, Bates ER, Berger PB, Clark DA, Cusma JT, Dehmer GJ, Kern MJ, Laskey WK, O'Laughlin MP, Oesterle S et al American College of Cardiology/Society for Cardiac Angiography and Interventions Clinical Expert Consensus Document on cardiac catheterization laboratory standards. A report of the American College of Cardiology Task Force on Clinical Expert Consensus Documents. J Am Coll Cardiol 2001; 37: 2170–2214

Berman DS, Hachamovitch R, Kiat H et al Incremental value of prognostic testing in patients with known or suspected ischemic heart disease: a basis for optimal utilization of exercise technetium-99m sestamibi myocardial perfusion single-photon emission computed tomography. J Am Coll Cardiol 1995; 26: 639–647

Beohar N et al Quantitative assessment of in-stents dimensions a comparison of 64 and 16 detector multislice computed tomography to intravascular ultrasound. Catheter Cardiovas Interv 2006; 68:8–10

Brown ER, Kronmal RA. Coronary calcium coverage score: determination, correlates, and predictive accuracy in the multiethnic study of atherosclerosis. Radiology 2008; 247(3): 669

Burkoff BW, Linker DT. Safety of intracoronary ultrasound data from a Multicenter European registry. Cather Cardiovasc Diagn 1996; 38:238–241

Cademartiri F et al Usefulness of 64-slice multislice computed tomography coronary angiography to assess in-stent restenosis. J Am Coll Cardiol 2007; 49:2204–2210

Campbell M. Natural history of coarctation of the aorta. Heart J 1970; 32:633–640

Carole A, Warnes MD The adult with congenital heart disease. Born to be bad? JACC 2005; 46(1):1–8

Carrascosa1 PM, Capuñay1 CM, Parodi2 JC, Padilla LT. General utilities of multislice tomography in the cardiac field. Herz 2003; 28:44–51

Chiurlia E et al Follow-up of coronary artery bypass graft patency by multislice computed tomography. Am J Cardiol 2005; 95:1094–1097

Cohen M, Fuster V, Steele PM et al Coarctation of the aorta. Long-term follow-up and prediction of outcome after surgical correction. Circulation 1989; 80:840–845

Dewey M, Laule M, Krug L, Schnapauff D, Rogalla P, Rutsch W, Hamm B, Lembcke A. Multisegment and halfscan reconstruction of 16-slice computed tomography for detection of coronary artery stenoses. Invest Radiol 2004; 39:223–229

Diamond GA, Staniloff HM, Forrester JS, Pollock BH, Swan HJ. Computer assisted diagnosis in the noninvasive evaluation of patients with suspected coronary artery disease. J Am Coll Cardiol 1983; 1:444–455

Gaspar T, Halon DA, Lewis, BS, Adawi S, Schliamser JE, Rubinshtein R. Diagnosis of coronary in-stent restenosis with multidetector row spiral computed tomography. J Am Coll Cardiol 2005; 46:1573–1579

Gibbons RJ, Abrams J, Chatterjee K, Daley J, Deedwania PC, Douglas JS, Ferguson TB Jr, Fihn SD, Fraker TD Jr, Gardin JM et al ACC/AHA 2002 guideline update for the management of patients with chronic stable angina – summary article: a report of the American College of Cardiology/American Heart Association Task Force on practice guidelines (Committee on the management of patients with chronic stable angina). J Am Coll Cardiol 2003; 41:159–168

Gibbons RJ, Balady GJ, Bricker JT et al ACC/AHA 2002 guideline update for exercise testing: summary article – a report of the American College of Cardiology/ American Heart Association task force on practice guidelines (committee to update the 1997 exercise testing guidelines). Circulation 2002; 106: 1883–1892

Giesler T, Baum U, Ropers D et al Noninvasive visualization of coronary arteries using contrastenhanced multidetector CT: influence of heart rate on image quality and stenosis detection. AJR Am J Roentgenol 2002; 179:911–916

Gilard M, Cornily JC, Pennec PY, Le Gal G, Nonent M, Mansourati J, Blanc JJ, Boschat J. Assessment of coronary artery stents by 16 slice computed tomography. Heart 2006; 92:58–61

Gómez-Jaume A. [Coronary aneurysms of the left anterior descending coronary artery and the right coronary artery after drug-eluting stent implantation]. Rev Esp Cardiol 2007; 60(9):992–997

Henneman MM et al Noninvasive evaluation with multislice computed tomography in suspected acute coronary syndrome plaque morphology on multislice computed tomography versus coronary calcium score. J Am Coll Cardiol 2008; 52(3):216–222

Hoffmann MH, Shi H, Schmid FT, Gelman H, Brambs H-J, Aschoff AJ. Noninvasive coronary imaging with MDCT in comparison to invasive conventional coronary angiography: a fast-developing technology. AJR Am J Roentgenol 2004; 182: 601–608

Hoffmann MH, Shi H, Schmitz BL, Schmid FT, Lieberknecht M, Schulze R, Ludwig B, Kroschel U, Jahnke N, Haerer W, Brambs HJ, Aschoff AJ. Noninvasive coronary angiography with multislice computed tomography. JAMA 2005; 293: 2471–2478

Hoffmann U et al Noninvasive assessment of plaque morphology and composition in culprit and stable lesions in acute coronary syndrome and stable lesions in stable angina by multidetector computed tomography. J Am Coll Cardiol 2006; 47(8):1665–1662

Hoffmann U, Hadvar J, Dunn E et al Is CT angiography ready for prime time? A meta-analysis. J Am Coll Cardiol 2004; 43(Suppl A):312A

Kaiser C, Bremerich J, Haller S, Brunner-La Rocca HP, Bongartz G, Pfisterer M, Buser P. Limited diagnostic yield of non-invasive coronary angiography by 16-slice multi-detector spiral computed tomography in routine patients referred for evaluation of coronary artery disease. Eur Heart J 2005; 26:1987–1992

Keane MG. Bicuspid aortic valves are associated with aortic dilatation out of proportion to coexistent valvular lesions. Circulation 2000; 102(suppl III):III35–III39

Kuettner A, Beck T, Drosch T et al Diagnostic accuracy of noninvasive coronary imaging using 16-detector slice spiral computed tomography with 188 ms temporal resolution. J Am Coll Cardiol 2005; 45:123–127

Kuettner A, Beck T, Drosch T, Kettering K, Heuschmid M, Burgstahler C, Claussen CD, Kopp AF, Schroeder S. Image quality and diagnostic accuracy of non invasive coronary imaging with 16 detector slice spiral computed tomography with 188 ms temporal resolution. Heart 2005; 91:938–941

Kuettner A, Beck T, Drosch T, Kettering K, Heuschmid M, Burgstahler C, Claussen CD, Kopp AF, Schroeder S. Diagnostic accuracy of noninvasive coronary imaging using 16-detector slice spiral computed tomography with 188 ms temporal resolution. J Am Coll Cardiol 2005; 45:123–127

Kuettner A, Trabold T, Schroeder S, Feyer A, Beck T, Brueckner A, Heuschmid M, Burgstahler C, Kopp AF, Claussen CD. Noninvasive detection of coronary lesions using 16-detector multislice spiral computed tomography technology: initial clinical results. J Am Coll Cardiol 2004; 44:1230–1237

Leber AW et al Accuracy of multidetector spiral CT in identifying and differentiating the composition of coronary atherosclerotic plaques. J Am Coll Cardiol 2004; 43:1241–1247

Ley S et al Preoperative assessment and follow up of congenital abnormalities of the pulmonary arteries using CT and MRI. Eur Radiol 2007; 17:151–162

Marano R et al Italian multicenter, prospective study to evaluate the negative predictive value of 16- and 64-slice MDCT imaging in patients scheduled for coronary angiography (NIMISCAD-Non Invasive Multicenter Italian Study for Coronary Artery Disease). Eur Radiol. 2009 May;19(5):1114–23. Epub 2008 Dec 17

Marco AS, Cordeiro MD et al Atherosclerotic plaque characterization by multidetector row computed tomography angiography. J Am Coll Cardiol 2006; 47:C40–C47

Manzke R, Grass M, Nielsen T, Shechter G, Hawkes D. Adaptive temporal resolution optimization in helical cardiac cone beam CT reconstruction. Med Phys 2003; 30:3072–3080

Martuscelli E, Romagnoli A, D'Eliseo A, Razzini C, Tomassini M, Sperandio M, Simonetti G, Romeo F. Accuracy of thin-slice computed tomography in the detection of coronary stenoses. Eur Heart J 2004; 25:1043–1048

Messika D et al Assessment of the mitral valve by MSCT. J Am Coll Cardiol 2006; 48:411–413

Mollet NR et al Value of preprocedure multislice computed tomographic coronary angiography to predict the outcome of percutaneous recanalization of chronic total occlusions. Am J Cardiol 2005; 15:95(2):240–243

Mollet NR, Cademartiri F, Krestin GP et al Improved diagnostic accuracy with 16-row multi-slice computed tomography coronary angiography. J Am Coll Cardiol 2005; 45:128–132

Mollet NR, Cademartiri F, Krestin GP, McFadden EP, Arampatzis CA, Serruys PW, de Feyter PJ. Improved diagnostic accuracy with 16-row multi-slice computed tomography coronary angiography. J Am Coll Cardiol 2005; 45:128–132

Motoyama S et al Multislice computed tomographic characteristics of coronary lesions in acute coronary syndromes. J Am Coll Cardiol 2007; 50(4):319–326

Nieman K, Cademartiri F, Lemos PA, Raaijmakers R, Pattynama PM, de Feyter PJ. Reliable noninvasive coronary angiography with fast submillimeter multislice spiral computed tomography. Circulation 2002; 106:2051–2054

Niemann K, Oudkerk M, Rensing B, van Ooijen P, Munne A, van Geuns RJ, de Feyter PJ. Coronary angiography with multislice computed tomography. Circulation 2001; 357:599–603

Nissen SE, Yock P. Intravascular ultrasound: novel pathophysiological insights and current clinical applications. Circulation 2001; 103:604–616

Oliver JM et al Risk factors for aortic complications in adults with coarctation of aorta. JACC 2004; 44:1641–1647

Otsuka M et al Utility of multislice computed tomography as a strategic tool for complex percutaneous coronary intervention. Catheter Cardiovasc Interv 2008; 71(4):490–503

Pannu HK et al Gated cardiac image of the aortic valve. J Compu Assist Tomograph 2006; 30:443–446

Pugliese F, Mollet MR et al Diagnostic accuracy of non-invasive 64-slice CT coronary angiography in patients with stable angina pectoris. Eur Radiol 2006; 16:575–582

Raff GL. Interpreting the evidence: How accurate is coronary computed tomography. J Cardiovasc Comput Tomogr 2007; 1:73–77

Raff GL et al Diagnostic accuracy of noninvasive coronary angiography using 64-slice spiral computed tomography. J Am Coll Cardiol 2005; 46(3):552–557

Rixe J, Achenbach S, Ropers D et al Assessment of coronary artery stent restenosis by 64-slice multi-detector computed tomography. Eur Heart J 2006; 27:2567–2572

Ropers D, Baum U, Pohle K, Anders K, Ulzheimer S, Ohnesorge B, Schlundt C, Bautz W, Daniel WG, Achenbach S. Detection of coronary artery stenoses with thin-slice multi-detector row spiral computed tomography and multiplanar reconstruction. Circulation 2003; 107:664–666

Rubinshtein R, Halon DA, Gaspar T, Jaffe R, Karkabi B, Flugelman MY, Kogan A, Shapira R, Peled N, Lewis BS. Usefulness of 64-slice cardiac computed tomographic angiography for diagnosing acute coronary syndromes and predicting clinical outcome in emergency department patients with chest pain of uncertain origin. Circulation 2007; 115(13): 1762–1768

Scanlon P, Faxon D, Audet A et al; Society for Cardiac Angiography and Interventions. ACC/AHA guidelines for coronary angiography: a report of the American College of Cardiology/American Heart Association Task Force on practice guidelines (committee on coronary angiography). J Am Coll Cardiol 1999; 33:1756–1824

Scanlon PJ, Faxon DP, Audet AM, Carabello B, Dehmer GJ, Eagle KA, Legako RD, Leon DF, Murray JA, Nissen SE et al ACC/AHA guidelines for coronary angiography. A report of the American College of Cardiology/American Heart Association Task Force on practice guidelines (Committee on Coronary Angiography). Developed in collaboration with the Society for Cardiac Angiography and Interventions. J Am Coll Cardiol 1999; 33:1756–1824

Schlosser T et al Noninvasive visualization of coronary artery bypass grafts using 16-detector row computed tomography. J Am Coll Cardiol 2004; 44:1224–1229

Schoenhagen P et al Non-invasive assessment plaque morphology and remodeling in mildly stenotic coronary stenosis Coron Artery Dis 2003; 14:459–462

Schroeder S, Kopp AF, Baumbach A et al Noninvasive detection and evaluation of atherosclerotic coronary plaques with multislice computed tomography. J Am Coll Cardiol 2001; 37: 1430–1435

Schuijf JD et al Feasibility of coronary stent imaging with multislice computed tomography. Eur J Radiol Extra 2004; 50: 59–62

Smuclovisky C, Baum S, Dhir M, Arora UK, McInnis P. Evaluation of patients with congenital coronary anomalies with cardiac CT angiography. South Florida Medical Imaging, Boca Raton, Florida, USA. University of Texas Health Science Center at San Antonio, TX, USA, 2006

Smuclovisky C, Baum S, Dhir M, Arora UK, McInnis P. Ealuation of patients post coronary bypass with cardiac CT angiography, South Florida Medical Imaging, Boca Raton, Florida, USA, 2006

Van Mieghem CA et al Multislice spiral computed tomography for the evaluation of stent patency after left main coronary artery stenting: a comparison with conventional coronary angiography and intravascular ultrasound. Circulation 2006; 114: 645–653

Vriend JWJ, Mulder BJM. Late complications in patients after repair of aortic coarctation. Implications for management. Int J Cardiol 2005; 101:399–406

Watkins M, Hesse B, Green C, Greenberg N, Manning M, Chaudhry E, Dauerman H, Garcia M. Detection of coronary artery stenosis using 40-channel computed tomography with multisegment reconstruction. Am J Cardiol 2007; 99(2):175–181

Yang TH, Kim DI et al Clinical characteristics of stent fracture after sirolimus-eluting stent implantation. Int J Cardiol 2009; 131:212–216

Echocardiography

2

Paola Kuschnir

Gustavo Avegliano, Marcelo Trivi, and Ricardo Ronderos (Contributors)

Introduction

From its first steps in the diagnosis of cardiovascular diseases, echocardiography imaging, such as M-mode, 2-D echocardiography and cardiovascular Doppler, has made tremendous advances until today. From primitive equipment that encouraged creativity and imagination, to 3-D echo, which shows structures the way surgeons see them during cardiac surgery, it has been an unthinkable journey for the pioneers in echocardiography.

Nowadays, echocardiography is the most widely used imaging technique for the diagnosis of cardiovascular diseases. This expansion was the result of a number of advantages such as its non-invasive low-risk nature, easy transportation of equipment, simplicity, and low cost. Moreover, there has been considerable improvement in image quality as a result of the development of transesophageal echocardiography and the technological advance of transthoracic transducers.

Echocardiography has contributed to the understanding and description of several cardiovascular diseases. Some paradigmatic examples are valvular diseases and hypertrophic and restrictive cardiomyopathies. Also the non-compaction of the left ventricular myocardium and Tako Tsubo syndrome are "echo diseases". The concept of mechanical dyssynchrony is mainly echocardiographic.

The Achilles' heel of echocardiography is that it is an explorer-dependent technique, which demands in-depth knowledge, the use of a well-defined methodology, and sound clinical correlation.

This chapter aims to show a series of pathologies that are seen in high-volume services, in order to enlighten those who have similar cases. All have been selected following a thorough learning approach and assessment protocols. We looked for cases where the diagnosis left no doubts.

Our goal is to show both the benefits of transthoracic and transesophageal echocardiography for different cardiovascular diseases and the usefulness of the wide range of available tools: 2D echo, conventional and tissue Doppler, contrast echo, 3D echo, etc. We also show further capabilities of the technique in the monitoring of invasive surgical and percutaneous procedures.

Finally, we focus on the relevance of echocardiography for the interpretation of patophysiological processes, clinical decision-making and prognosis.

Case 2.1
Apical Myocardial Hypertrophy

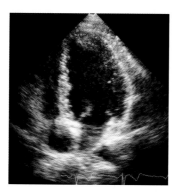

Fig. 2.1.1

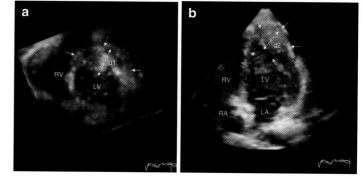

Fig. 2.1.2

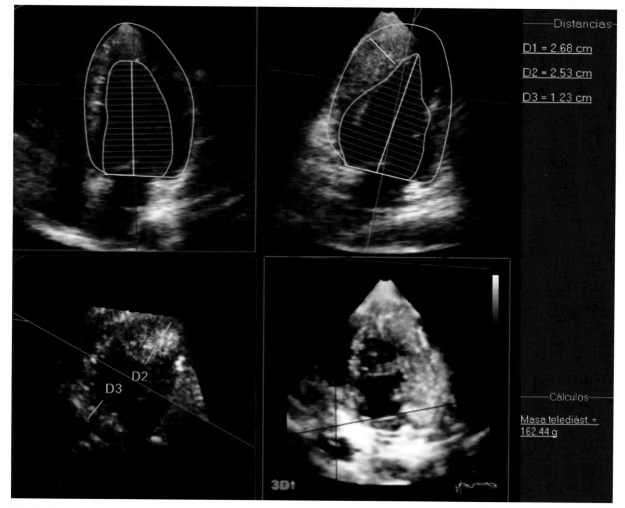

Fig. 2.1.3

A 29-year-old man with prior history of smoking presented to the emergency department complaining of oppressive chest pain. An electrocardiogram (ECG) showed asymmetric negative T waves in leads I, aV_L, V_2 to V_4. Cardiac enzymes were normal. The patient underwent noninvasive nuclear imagining that ruled out cardiac ischemia. Transthoracic bidimensional (2DE) and real-time 3D imaging (RT3DE) echocardiogram were performed.

Comments

Apical hypertrophic cardiomyopathy (HCM) is characterized by localized hypertrophy at the apical left ventricular segments. A pathognomonic feature of apical HCM is the presence of deep symmetric T-wave inversion in the anterior precordial leads. The presence of these latter ECG changes frequently suggests its diagnosis in the asymptomatic form of the disease. Symptomatic patients present with typical (16%) or atypical (14%) angina, palpitations (10%), dyspnea on exertion (6%), or syncopal episodes (6%). This form of HCM usually has a benign course and a good long-term prognosis. Nevertheless, its overt ECG changes mandate clinical rule-out of severe epicardial coronary stenosis by noninvasive imaging.

Cardiac magnetic resonance imaging (MRI) is currently the most sensitive and specific available technique for the diagnosis of apical HCM. MRI has an excellent accuracy for the measurement of myocardial thickness, providing an adequate assessment of the degree and extension of myocardial hypertrophy. Still, due to cost constraints, routine screening usually starts with 2DE with harmonic imaging. As a second step, further evaluation with either contrast 2DE or MRI should be followed, especially in cases with high clinical suspicion or poor echo window.

RT3DE enables precise heart slicing through the apex. The latter is particularly difficult to perform with 2D echocardiography due to foreshortening. Furthermore, utilization of RT3DE allows acquisition of any given slice across the left ventricle, thus obtaining a better morphological characterization of the HCM (i.e., myocardial thickness and distribution) than standard 2DE.

Findings

Figure 2.1.1 2DE shows a nondiagnostic image at the apex.

Figure 2.1.2 Left ventricular volume imaging is obtained by RT3DE. (a) Note the presence of segmental myocardial hypertrophy at the apical level. RT3DE apical view, which shows maximal myocardial thickness at the anterior and lateral apical segments (*arrows*), d2 = 26 mm. (b) Four-chamber view eliminating the inferior heart region. Note the disproportional hypertrophy at the apical segment of the lateral wall (*arrows*), d1 = 27 mm.

Figure 2.1.3 RT3DE. Multiplanar image shows an asymmetric distribution of hypertrophy. Note the measurement of myocardial thickness and quantification of the left ventricular mass.

Case 2.2
■
Severe Mitral Insufficiency Secondary to Papillary Muscle Rupture

A 74-year-old woman with a history of arterial hypertension and essential thrombocythemia presented to the emergency room complaining of intermittent chest pain and severe dyspnea for 5 days. On arrival, the patient had bilateral pulmonary edema in addition to III/VI systolic murmur that radiated to the axilla suggestive of mitral regurgitation. ECG revealed mild ST-segment elevation in leads DII and aV$_F$. Lab results showed high platelet count (960,000/ml) and mild troponine I elevation (1.95 ng/ml). The patient underwent cardiac catheterization that showed only a mild lesion (20%) on the mid-portion of the arterial circumflex coronary artery. A Doppler echocardiogram was performed to further elucidate the etiology of this left-sided heart failure.

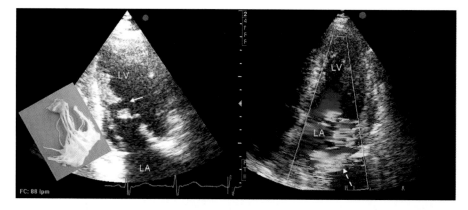

Fig. 2.2.1

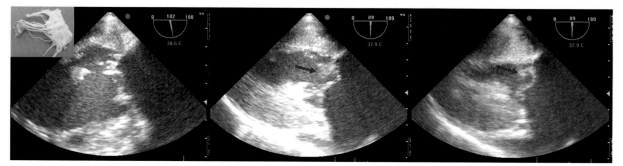

Fig. 2.2.2

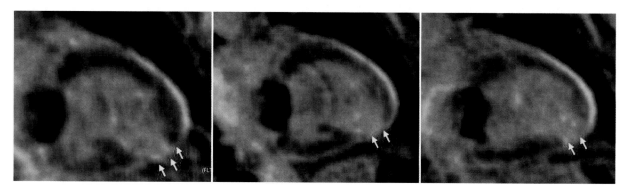

Fig. 2.2.3

Ischemic mitral regurgitation (MR) is due to either myocardial ischemia or infarction in the absence of primary structural valve abnormality. Moderate to severe ischemic MR during the acute phase of myocardial infarction is associated with a poor short- and long-term clinical outcome.

Ischemic MR is classified according to its presentation and pathophysiology: type I and II are due to acute ischemic injury linked to papillary muscle dysfunction (type I) or rupture (type II). Type III is related to fibrosis or sclerosis of the papillary muscle, likely due to an old myocardial infarction. Type IV is due to loss of the normal left ventricular architecture following a large myocardial infarction. Type III and IV have a more insidious presentation following an acute myocardial infarction than type I and II have.

An accurate understanding of the culprit mechanism of MR is of utmost importance in order to provide the best therapy for each individual case. Thus, type I ischemic MR may only require myocardial revascularization, while type II will definitely undergo either surgical mitral valve repair or replacement.

Transthoracic echocardiography (TTE) is very useful for the diagnosis and quantification of ischemic MR as well as the evaluation of the mechanism responsible for the disease. Furthermore, it enables an estimate of pulmonary arterial pressure and quantification of left ventricular systolic function. In our experience, mitral valve evaluation requires further imaging with transesophageal echocardiography (TEE), since its higher spatial resolution provides detailed information regarding the valve and its apparatus. In summary, we studied a peculiar case of acute myocardial infarction with nonsevere coronary stenosis at the time of catheterization complicated with posterior papillary rupture and severe acute MR.

Comments

Findings

Figure 2.2.1 *Left:* 2D TTE two-chamber view. In this image posterior papillary muscle rupture is clearly demonstrated (*continuous arrow*). Anatomic correlation of papillary muscle rupture is observed. In this particular case, both papillary muscles provide cords to both mitral leaflets. Note cusp rupture of the anterior leaflet, which presents abnormal closure. In the right image, color Doppler (four-chamber view) imaging reveals the presence of a mitral regurgitation jet (*dotted arrow*) coursing laterally to the left atrial wall.

Figure 2.2.2 Transgastric 90° TEE view. *Left:* image recorded at diastole showing the flail cusp of the posterior papillary muscle inside the left ventricle. *Center:* image at mid-systole showing posterior cusp folding to the ventricular side of the mitral valve. *Right:* image at late systole showing complete folding of the cusp and a striking prolapse of the anterior leaflet responsible for the presence of mitral valve insufficiency. Red arrows show the cusp of the papillary muscle.

Figure 2.2.3 Two-chamber DE-MRI view performed after surgical valve replacement, revealing transmural hyperintensity localized at the level of the mid- and apical segments of the inferior wall (*arrows*) with partial involvement of the posterior papillary muscle. Note artifact generated by the mitral valve prosthesis.

Case 2.3
■
Noncompacted Cardiomyopathy

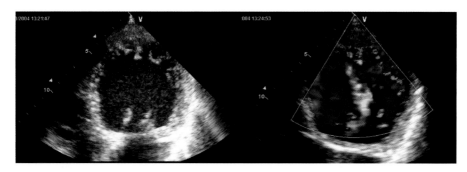

Fig. 2.3.1

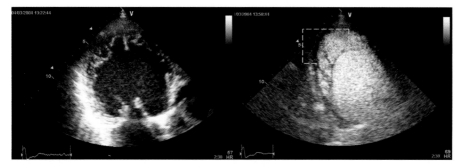

Fig. 2.3.2

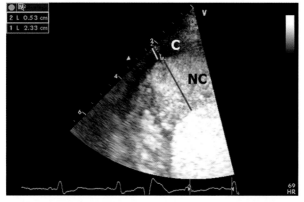

Fig. 2.3.3

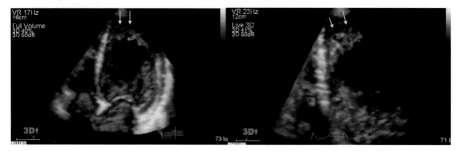

Fig. 2.3.4

A 37-year-old man, with no coronary risk factors, presented to our office complaining of palpitations and dyspnea on minimal exertion. An ECG demonstrated complete left bundle branch block. A chest X-ray showed cardiomegaly without any signs of venocapilar hypertension. Contrast and Doppler echocardiograms were performed to elucidate patient's cardiac condition.

Comments

Noncompaction cardiomyopathy (NCCM) is a recently characterized cardiomyopathy in which ventricular myocardial compactation fails to occur during fetal development. In NCCM, multiple large trabecules plus intertrabecular recesses are observed deep in the myocardium, especially at the apical segments. Imaging diagnostic criteria for NCCM require an area of noncompacted/compacted myocardium >2.3.

Various imaging techniques provide adequate sensitivity for the diagnosis of NCCM, and there are some cases when combining different techniques may be complementary. Bidimensional transthoracic echocardiography (2DE) is adequate for quantification of noncompacted myocardial regions, while visualization of compacted regions is cumbersome. Quantification of compacted myocardium with 2DE is greatly improved with the use of contrast agents. The author believes that contrast echocardiographic assessment of noncompacted/compacted myocardial index is best performed with zoom during diastole in regions where papillary muscles will not overlap (i.e., apical, latero-apical, and inferior-lateral).

Additional data can be obtained regarding the distribution and localization of non-compacted myocardial areas with RT3DE. Currently, MRI, due to its excellent spatial and tissue resolution, represents the most detailed and precise imaging technique for the assessment of NCCM. In addition, MRI is particularly useful in patients with mild form of the disease or in patients with poor echo window. Multidetector computed tomography of the heart also conveys myocardial morphological information, and can thus be an option especially in patients with suspected coronary artery disease. In summary, all the above-mentioned imaging techniques provide reliable data regarding the degree of trabeculation in the left ventricle. Nonetheless, NCCM diagnosis should not be performed with only one isolated measurement. Imaging data derived from morphological myocardial quantification and the assessment of global left ventricular function often need correlation with the patient's clinical condition and, in some cases, familial evaluation (i.e., genetic testing) in order to obtain an accurate diagnosis.

Findings

Figure 2.3.1 *Left*: 2DE, apical four-chamber view revealing large trabecules and deep intertrabecular recesses in the left ventricle. *Right*: Color flow Doppler signal filling these recesses.

Figure 2.3.2 *Left*: 2DE, apical three-chamber view demonstrates multiple deep trabecule formation inside the myocardium, which clearly defines the noncompacted myocardium. *Right*: The compacted area is visualized with contrast agent administration. The *square* (zoom) demarcates the studied myocardial region.

Figure 2.3.3 Contrast echo (with zoom) performed during diastole. Note how the compacted myocardium acquires a dark color, improving its visualization. The noncompacted/compacted myocardial index was greater than 2.5.

Fig 2.3.4 Left ventricular volume imaging is obtained by RT3DE. Showing the non compaction at the apical segments with RT3DE. *Left*: Four-chamber view eliminating the inferior heart region. Note the apical hipertrabeculation (*arrows*). *Right*: the same image with zoom.

Case 2.4

■

Right Atrial Tumor

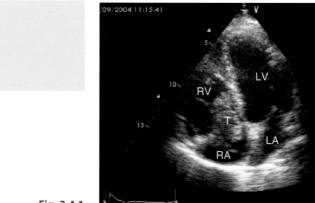

Fig. 2.4.1

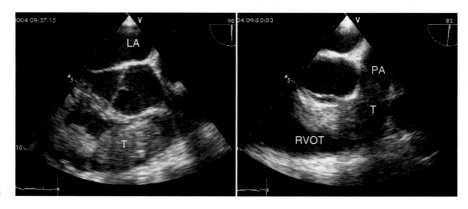

Fig. 2.4.2

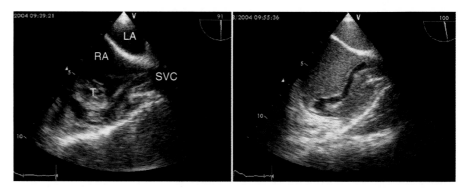

Fig. 2.4.3

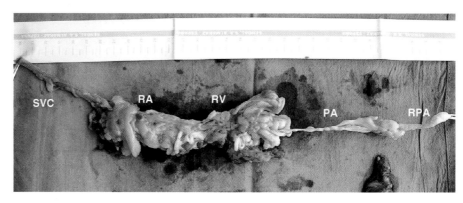

Fig. 2.4.4

A 38-year-old man with a prior history of testicular cancer presented to the emergency room with worsening dyspnea. One year prior to admission, he was diagnosed with metastatic non-seminomatous germ-cell tumor involving the lungs, the mediastinum, and the retroperitoneum. The patient underwent right orchiectomy and chemotherapy followed by surgical metastatic tissue resection, and remained asymptomatic until 1 week prior to this admission when he started feeling short of breath. Lung scan was performed and it revealed pulmonary embolisms in the mid and inferior right lobes. Then an echocardiogram was performed.

Comments

Primary cardiac tumors are infrequent. Benign mixomas account for half of all primary tumors. On the other hand, metastatic tumor involvement of the heart is much more common than primary cardiac tumors. In autopsy reports of patients with disseminated neoplasm, metastasis to the heart was found in 10–20% of the cases. Malignant melanoma most often involves the heart, followed by germ-cell tumors [e.g., metastasis to the heart was found in 38% of the necropsies performed in 100 patients with germ-cell tumors]. Transthoracic (TTE) and transesophageal (TEE) echocardiography are very instrumental in the morphological evaluation of cardiac masses and continues to be the first imaging techniques to be used in the presence of cardiac signs or symptoms potentially related to cardiac masses. TTE is readily available and offers sufficient spatial resolution plus adequate real-time imaging at low cost. Furthermore, its use provides clinically relevant information regarding valve function and the degree of hemodynamic compromise. Therefore, TTE represents the first imaging diagnostic step when dealing with cardiac masses. TEE enables a more detailed assessment of the size, mobility, and anchoring area of the tumor as well as its level of infiltration in cardiac structures. Magnetic resonance imaging (MRI) offers further details regarding tissue characterization and degree of infiltration of the tumor (e.g., pericardium and adjacent structures). Still, pathological confirmation is mandatory in all patients presenting with cardiac masses. This particular case shows a patient with right atrial tumor, found to be metastasis of a non-seminomatous germ-cell tumor.

Findings

Figure 2.4.1 TTE. Apical four-chamber view revealing a large mass with irregular borders through the tricuspid valve. *RV* right ventricle; *RA* right atrium; *T* tumor; *LV* left ventricle; *LA* left atrium.

Figure 2.4.2 TEE at the level of cavas. *Left*: Note a large tumoral mass that involves the superior vena cava as a low echogenic pedunculated mass, which is also observed in the right atrium as a multilobulated mass. *Right*: Contrast TEE unveils the vascular pedicle of the tumor (i.e., the contrast agent diffuses into the vascular region of the tumor and clearly delineates the peduncular area).

Figure 2.4.3 TEE. *Left*: 90° image revealing a mass that passes through the right ventricular outflow tract. *Right* image: the mass reaches the pulmonary artery trunk. *RVOT* right ventricular outflow tract; *PA* pulmonary artery trunk.

Figure 2.4.4 Macroscopic image of a surgically excised mass. Note the exact position of each portion of the mixoma within the heart and adjacent vascular structures. *SVC* superior vena cava; *RA* right atrium; *RV* right ventricle; *PA* pulmonary artery (trunk); *RPA* right pulmonary artery.

Case 2.5
■
Lateral Left Ventricular Wall Rupture Following Acute Myocardial Infarction

A 79-year-old man with a history of chronic obstructive pulmonary disease due to smoking and a long-standing history of coronary artery disease requiring surgical myocardial revascularization (left internal mammary artery to left anterior descending coronary artery and a vein graft to right coronary artery) 10 years prior to this admission presented with new onset of resting chest pain. ECG was normal. Cardiac catheterization showed patency of both grafts, left anterior descending coronary artery with proximal total occlusion, first diagonal with an 80% stenosis and first marginal of circumflex with a 90% stenosis. The patient underwent stenting of both diagonal and marginal lesions and remained asymptomatic for 76 h when he had a syncopal episode associated with severe bradicardia with fast recovery followed by complaints of chest pain. ECG showed diffuse ST-segment elevation. After 10 min, symptoms abated and ECG changes resolved. A diagnostic echocardiogram was performed.

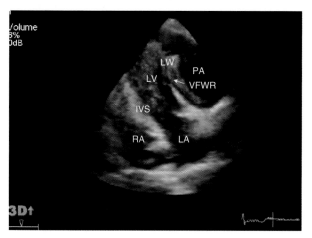

Fig. 2.5.3

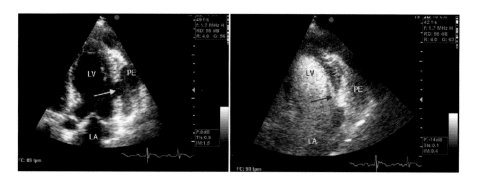

Fig. 2.5.1

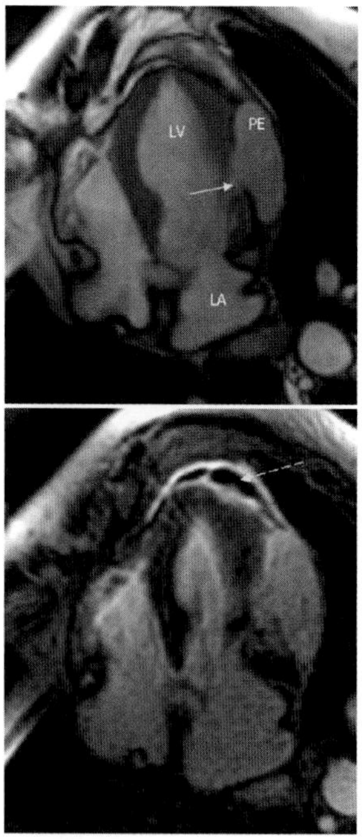

Fig. 2.5.2 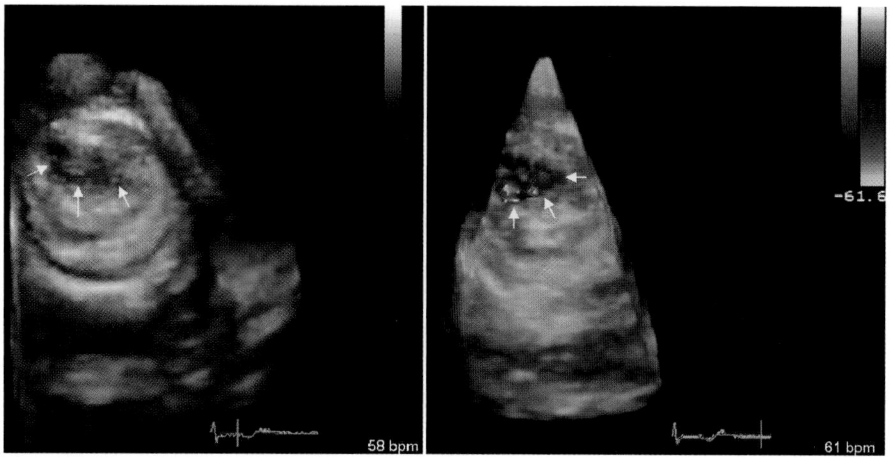   **Fig. 2.5.4**

Lateral left ventricular wall rupture (LWR) is a rare complication following acute myocardial infarction (AMI; 3–5%), reaching 10–25% in autopsy of AMI patients. After cardiogenic shock, LWR constitutes the most common cause of in-hospital death in AMI patients. Around 40% of all LWR occur during the first 24 h and 85% within the first week. It is frequently associated with advanced age, female gender, systemic arterial hypertension, absence of preinfarction angina, and no visible collaterals during catheterization. Diagnosis is suspected in patients with severe hypotension, extreme bradicardia, or cardiac arrest with electrical mechanical dissociation. Rupture is confirmed with echocardiographic evidence of a large pericardial effusion, with echoes suggestive of hemopericardium. As in the present case, patients with prior history of cardiac surgery may experience self-limited myocardial rupture with prompt sealing due to pericardial adhesions, resulting in a pseudoaneurysm. The development of a pseudoaneurysm after an AMI is exceedingly low and its natural evolution is unknown.

Usually, bidimensional and contrast TTE suffices for purposes of clinical diagnosis. On the other hand, real-time 3D echocardiography (RT3DE) gives greater anatomical and functional information than TTE and emerges as an exceptional imaging tool prior to surgical intervention. In the present case, 76 h following the intervention, LWR was observed likely due to a small infarction at the lateral left ventricular wall possibly because of the marginal lesion. Our patient refused surgery and was followed up clinically. Eighteen months later, RT3DE showed a consolidated pseudoaneurysm.

Figure 2.5.1 TTE (acute phase). *Left*: Note the rupture at the mid-portion of the lateral left ventricular wall (*arrow*) and a localized pericardial effusion adjacent to the lateral wall. *Right*: Contrast TTE. Note contrast filling of the pericardium and opacification of a parallel cavity, in relation to the left ventricle, with systolic and diastolic flow through the rupture.

Figure 2.5.2 MRI. *Left*: Cine-MRI (SSFP) at four-chamber view. Note the LWR (*arrow*) and localized pericardial effusion. *Right*: Delayed enhancement-MRI (inversion-recovery) following gadolinium administration. Presence of thrombotic pericardial adhesions in the apical region (*dashed arrow*). Absence of late enhancement (related to the complete loss of tissue compatible with a small transmural myocardial infarction). *LV* left ventricle; *LA* left atrium; *PE* pericardial effusion.

Figure 2.5.3 RT3DE performed at 18 months from the event. Full ventricular volume image revealing a consolidated pseudoaneurysm and the rupture area at the mid-portion of the left lateral ventricular wall (*arrow*). LV left ventricle; LA left atrium; RA right atrium; IVS interventricular septum; LW lateral wall; PA pseudoaneurysm; VFWR ventricular free wall rupture.

Figure 2.5.4 Three-dimensional echocardiogram. *Left*: Full 3D volume processed image. View of the lateral wall from the pseudoaneurysm (the *darkest area* demarcated by the *arrows* indicates the rupture area). *Right*: With color flow Doppler during diastole, note three *small points* suggesting regurgitant flow from the pseudoaneurysm to the left ventricular wall.

Case 2.6
![black square]

Traumatic Rupture of the Tricuspid Valve

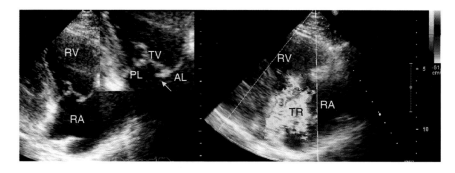

Fig. 2.6.1

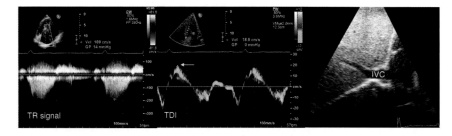

Fig. 2.6.2

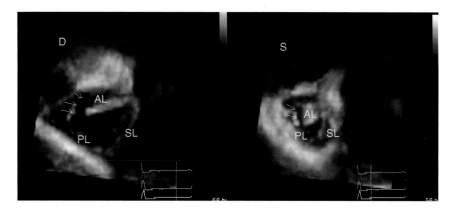

Fig. 2.6.3

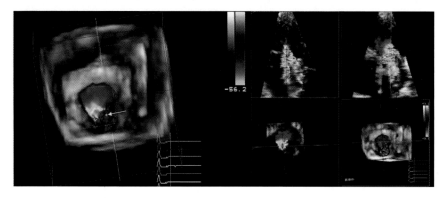

Fig. 2.6.4

A 39-year-old asymptomatic man is referred for an echocardiogram due to the presence of cardiac systolic murmur. He has no prior significant medical history, except for a motor vehicle accident (MVA) 3 years earlier.

Comments

MVA accounts for most cases of traumatic rupture of the tricuspid valve. Valve rupture during an MVA is generated by an abrupt deceleration coupled with an increase in right-side cardiac pressures (Valsalva maneuver and thorax compression). The most frequent rupture site is the tendinous cords, followed by the anterior papillary muscle and tear or detachment of the anterior leaflet. During the acute phase of an MVA, life-threatening lesions to the head, thorax, or abdomen are of most clinical relevance. Thus, accurate cardiac diagnosis during MVA is cumbersome, especially when dealing with discrete or moderate valve lesions. Diagnosis of tricuspid valve rupture is usually delayed, due to its mild clinical course. Echocardiography plays an important role in the diagnosis, follow-up, and surgical indication in patients with tricuspid valve rupture. Knowledge of right ventricle diameter and function in addition to data regarding the systemic venous circulation is of interest prior to tricuspid valve surgery. Performing color and tissue Doppler echocardiography plus cardiac magnetic resonance imaging represents the best combination prior to surgery. Finally, real-time 3D echocardiography (RT3DE) emerges as a novel useful imaging tool, offering a detailed anatomic and functional assessment of the tricuspid valve – useful data that may assess valve repair feasibility and decide the most appropriate repair technique.

Findings

Figure 2.6.1 TTE. *Left*: longitudinal view of the right ventricle during systole. Note the lineal image at mid-portion of the tricuspid anterior leaflet (*arrow*) compatible with cord rupture. Nevertheless, it is interesting how central coaptation is not lost. *Right side*: color Doppler image showing severe tricuspid regurgitation. *RA* right atrium; *RV* right ventricle; *PV* posterior valve; *AV* anterior valve; *TR* tricuspid regurgitation.

Figure 2.6.2 *From left to right*. Note the curve of tricuspid insufficiency without evidence of pulmonary arterial hypertension. RV function by tissue Doppler imaging was normal with a tricuspid annular systolic velocity >12 cm/seg (*arrow*), and inferior vena cava with normal inspiratory collapse suggests normal right-side cardiac and venous pressures despite volume overload.

Figure 2.6.3 RT3DE: Postprocessed full volume image. Tricuspid valve is viewed from the RV. *Left*: (diastole) Note a tear at the body of the anterior leaflet (*arrow*) and not at the chord, as suggested by bidimensional echo. The tear is observed from the free border to the annulus. *Right*: (systole) tricuspid valve is closed and folded. Note the persistence of lineal image indicative of anterior leaflet rupture (*arrow*).

Figure 2.6.4 RT3DE. *Left*: full volume color Doppler of the tricuspid valve from the RV, showing a regurgitant orifice through the rupture (*arrow*). *Right*: 3D multiplanar quantification of the three-dimensional regurgitant orifice, vena contracta, and hemisphere.

Case 2.7
◼
Complicated Type B Aortic Dissection

A 61-year-old man with history of hypertension was admitted with acute aortic dissection type B. During his stay in the CCU, he complained of post-pandrial abdominal pain. Transesophageal echocardiogram (TEE) demonstrated compression of both celiac trunk

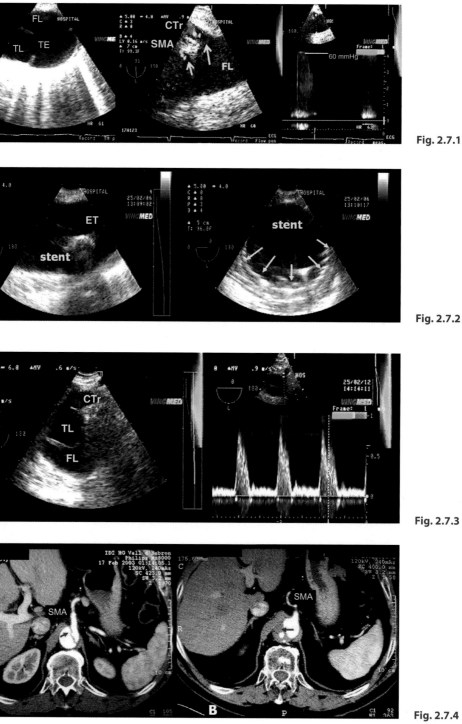

Fig. 2.7.1

Fig. 2.7.2

Fig. 2.7.3

Fig. 2.7.4

(CTr) and superior mesenteric artery (SMA). Due to the presence of mesenteric ischemia as a complication of a type B aortic dissection, we proceeded with endovascular closure of the entry tear guided by imaging techniques with good results.

Acute aortic dissection (AAD) is the most frequent form of acute aortic syndromes and is also associated with the worst clinical outcome. Its mortality surpasses 60% during the first week if adequate treatment is not instituted fast. Besides cardiac complications, intimal dissection process can obstruct the ostium of several aortic arterial branches, with great potential for ischemia in a number of organs. Organ ischemia distally from the aortic dissection is frequently observed (30%). In the international registry of aortic dissection (IRAD), mesenteric ischemia was detected in 5.4% of the cases and it was associated with a high mortality risk. Early treatment of complicated dissections is crucial for patients' clinical course and long-term prognosis. Therefore, early and accurate diagnosis of arterial branch obstruction is needed in order to select the best therapeutic approach.

During an acute aortic syndrome, TEE allows rapid evaluation (≤15 min), at the patient's bedside or at the operating room, enabling an adequate monitoring of the patient's hemodynamics. TEE diagnostic sensitivity and specificity for the detection of aortic dissection is similar to other imaging techniques, providing location, size, and flow of the entry tear in addition to the degree of aortic insufficiency or presence of pericardial effusion/tamponade. In comparison with other imaging techniques, aortic arterial branch visualization by TEE is difficult, especially in the abdominal aorta. However, in centers with significant expertise accurate assessment of all abdominal aortic branches with TEE is feasible and provides complementary information to that obtained by computed tomography.

Comments

Findings

Figure 2.7.1 TEE. *Left*: transversal 0° view at the level of the proximal portion of the descending aorta proximally, where a large entry tear is observed. *Center*: longitudinal 93° view at the level of the CTr and SMA. Note the compression of both aortic branches secondary to intimal displacement due to elevated pressure at the false lumen (FL). In this image, the FL covers almost the entire aortic lumen and turbulence is clearly observed at the ostium of both aortic abdominal branches (*arrow*). *Right*: continuous Doppler signal at the level of the ostium of CTr demonstrating a 65 mmHg translational gradient compatible with severe obstruction. ET: entry tear, FL: false lumen, TL: true lumen, CTr: celiac trunck, SMA, superior mesenteric artery.

Figure 2.7.2 TEE monitoring during percutanous closure of the entry tear (ET). *Right*: 0° view of the aortic arch distally at the level of the entry tear showing correct placement of the stent prior to deployment. *Left*: similar image following stent deployment showing adequate stent apposition (*arrows*).

Figure 2.7.3 Quantification of CTr and SMA decompression. *Left*: transversal 0° view at the level of CTr, showing both patent branches with normal flow. *Right*: pulsed Doppler revealing normalization of systolic velocities with no significant gradient at the level of CTr and SMA (*arrows*).

Figure 2.7.4 *Left*: image taken prior to stent deployment showing compression of the SMA by the FL (*arrow*). *Right*: control image following EP closure. Note aortic and partial thrombosis of FL (*arrow*).

Case 2.8
■
Aortic Mobile Thrombosis

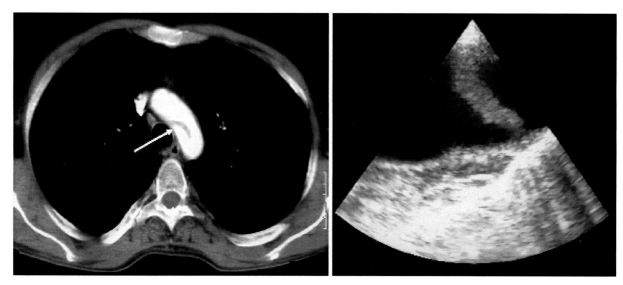

Fig. 2.8.1

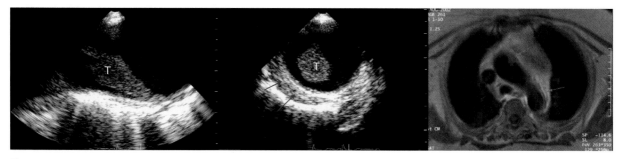

Fig. 2.8.2

We study two men who experienced acute limb ischemia. The first case is a 50-year-old patient with a history of dyslipidemia and new onset of upper left extremity ischemia, in which a computed tomography (CT) of the thorax was interpreted as aortic dissection at the arch level. The second case is an 80-year-old patient with low left extremity ischemia due to an embolic event in the clinical scenario of inflammation. Both cases underwent transesophageal echocardiogram (TEE).

Comments

Acute peripheral arterial ischemia may be the first manifestation of acute aortic dissection.

The presence of mobile aortic thrombosis is quite rare and is usually related to either complicated (i.e., ulcerated or debris accumulation) aortic plaques or to aortic aneurysms. Although rare, patients with nondilated otherwise normal aortas may develop an isolated aortic thrombus. In addition, the presence of aortic vasculitis can be unmasked by the detection of an aortic thrombus. Aortic thrombosis, particularly when the thrombus is mobile, is frequently associated with peripheral arterial embolism and may be mistaken for aortic dissection by some imaging techniques. Correct diagnosis is crucial because management differs in both entities.

As shown in the first case, TEE allows morphological characterization of the aortic wall and thrombus and rules out aortic dissection. The patient was started on antiplatelet and anticoagulant medications and thrombus regressed after 3 months. In the second case, mobile aortic thrombosis was in the context of vasculitis. The patient was diagnosed with giant cell arteritis (confirmed by temporal artery biopsy). The use of magnetic resonance imaging (MRI) in the second case was instrumental, showing inflammatory areas on the aortic wall, which helped obtain an accurate diagnosis.

Findings

Figure 2.8.1 (Case 1); *Right*: CT shows a linear image in the aortic arch (*arrow*) misdiagnosed as aortic dissection. Thrombus formation was interpreted as thrombosed intimal flap. *Left*: TEE reveals a 30-mm-long pedunculated thrombus in the aortic arch (patient 1).

Figure 2.82 (Case 2); TEE. *Left* and *center*: note a large pedunculated image with low echogenicity indicative of aortic thrombosis. The aortic vasculitic region presented thickening of the media layer and overt separation between adventitia and intima layers (*arrows*). *Right*: contrast MRI revealed a hyperintense signal suggestive of acute aortic inflammatory changes.

Case 2.9
■
Severe Mitral Insufficiency Secondary to Rupture of Posterior Leaflet

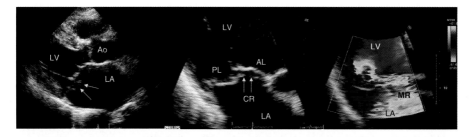

Fig. 2.9.1

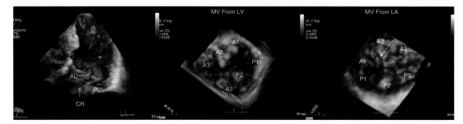

Fig. 2.9.2

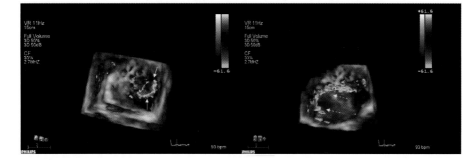

Fig. 2.9.3

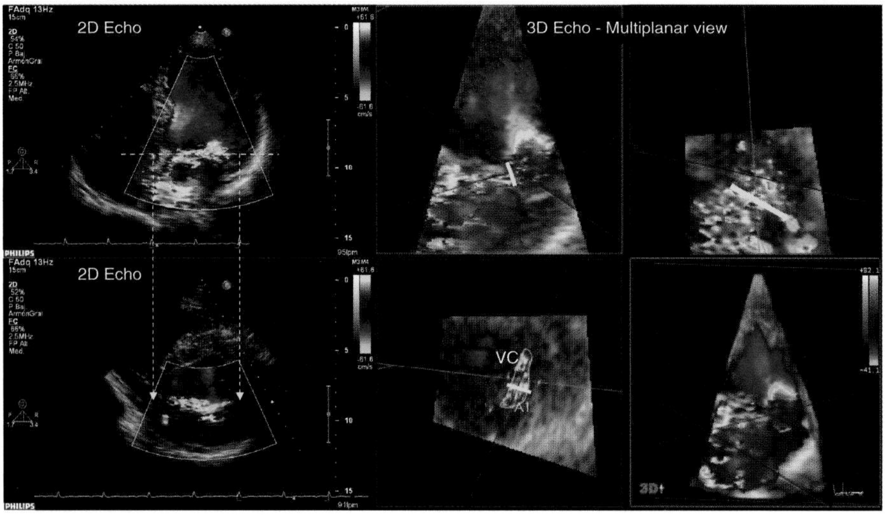

Fig. 2.9.4

A 52-year-old man, with no coronary risk factors, presented to our office complaining of dyspnea on exertion and palpitations. A systolic murmur was detected on auscultation and the patient underwent echocardiogram evaluation.

Mitral valve prolapse (MVP) has been described as the most common cardiac valvular abnormality in developed countries and the leading cause of mitral valve surgery for isolated mitral regurgitation (MR). Bidimensional echocardiography (2DE) is the most utilized imaging tool for diagnosing mitral valve disease, especially mitral valve prolapse. Occasionally, chordae tendinae of either the anterior or posterior mitral valve leaflet or both spontaneously rupture. Early detection and close surveillance of flail mitral valve is paramount due to its rapid progression to severe MR. Mitral valve repair is expected to provide better outcome than valve replacement, and requires a thorough understanding of mitral valve morphology. Echocardiographic evaluation is vital in order to determine the best timing for valve surgery. Conventional and color Doppler 2DE represents the first diagnostic tool for the diagnosis, quantification, and follow-up of flail mitral valve disease. In surgical candidates, transesophageal echocardiography (TEE) improves visualization of the valve and its apparatus, providing valuable data to gauge mitral valve repair feasibility and to evaluate surgical results. The emergence of real-time 3D echocardiography (RT3DE), either transthoracic or TEE, allows 3D reconstruction of the entire valve and its apparatus, which is a major improvement when compared to bidimensional images. RT3DE offers a great deal of morphological and functional information that helps understand different pathological mechanisms and plan an appropriate surgical strategy.

Figure 2.9.1 TTE 2DE. *Left*: paraesternal longitudinal view showing prolapse and eversion of the posterior leaflet (*arrows*). *Center*: three-chamber apical view with zoom. Note eversion of the posterior leaflet with rupture of the chordae (*arrows*). *Right*: three-chamber apical view with color Doppler image showing the origin of the regurgitant jet at the rupture site. *LV* left ventricle; *Ao* aorta; *LA* left atrium; *PL* posterior leaflet; *AL* leaflet; *CR* chordae rupture; *MR* mitral regurgitation.

Figure 2.9.2 RT3DE. *Left*: full volume four-chamber view in systole. Posterior oblique view revealing CR and eversion of PL. *Center*: zoom 3D image from LV. Note how the P2 segment is moving away to the LA. *Right*: view from LA in systole, clearly demonstrating the ruptured segment (P2 moving to the LA). Note ruptured chordae inside the LA (*arrow*).

Figure 2.9.3 Color Doppler flow on RT3DE. *Left*: LV viewed through a hemisphere (*arrow*). Note the regurgitant orifice that is initiated between P2-A2 segments. *Right*: view of the LA through the regurgitant jet. Note the coanda-effect at the anterior wall of the LA (*arrows*).

Figure 2.9.4 Color Doppler flow on TEE 2DE. *Left*: note the highly eccentric shape of the regurgitant jet traveling from the PL to the inter-auricular septum. Due to its eccentricity, exact estimation of its origin is cumbersome with 2DE. *Right*: color Doppler on RT3DE enabling visualization and quantification of the regurgitant jet in three different spatial planes at each moment of the cardiac cycle. Note how the vena contracta diameter differs according to the spatial plane used due to its elliptical shape.

Case 2.10
■
Endomyocardial Fibrosis Secondary to a Hypereosinophilic Syndrome

A 57-year-old male complained of progressive dyspnea for almost a year and was referred for further evaluation of his heart failure. The patient had a long-standing history of parasitic infection and hypereosinophilia (>1,500/ml).

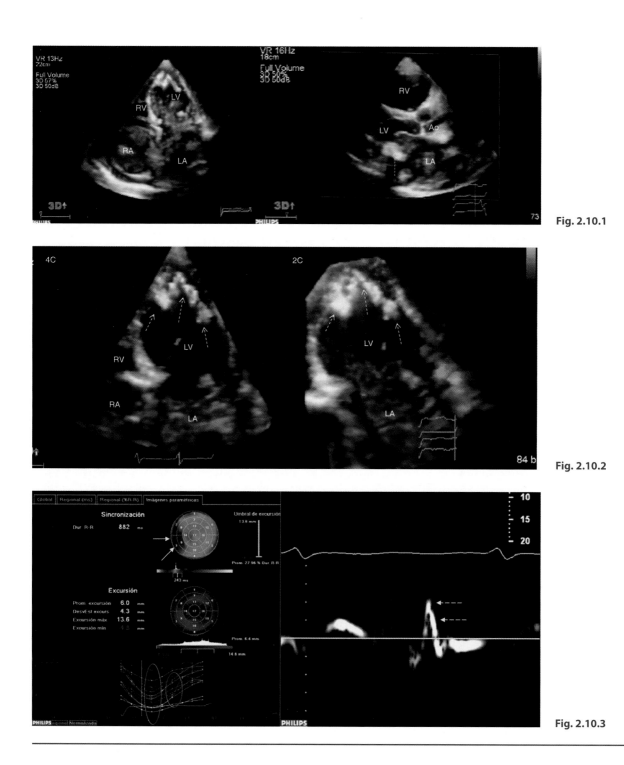

Fig. 2.10.1

Fig. 2.10.2

Fig. 2.10.3

Hypereosinophilic syndromes include endomyocardial fibrosis and Loeffler's endocarditis. These diseases are characterized by direct myocardial damage produced by eosinophilic cytotoxicity. Loeffler's endocarditis is part of an idiopathic hypereosinophilic syndrome. Endomyocardial fibrosis is endemic in African regions, India, and South America, and it is linked to parasitic infection. Endomyocardial fibrosis is usually due to the presence of dead parasites within the myocardium that provoke an inflammatory reaction and fibrosis. Myocardial microscopic evaluation shows intense fibrosis at the endocardium, especially at the apical regions of both right and left ventricles, obliterating both apexes. In addition, fibrosis may involve subvalvular tricuspid and mitral apparatus.

In the first phase of the disease, thrombus at the apexes may be visualized, followed by intense apical fibrosis and even calcification in some cases. These changes translate into alterations in ventricular filling, however, with still normal ventricular filling pressures and mild or absent clinical expression. During a later phase, fibrosis worsens resulting in a severe ventricular restrictive pattern and overt diastolic heart failure (left-side, right-side, or biventricular).

Echocardiography allows the direct diagnosis of the presence of small ventricles and dilated atriums. Color and tissue Doppler echo helps evaluate the patient's hemodynamic pattern and the degree of improvement with the instituted medical therapy.

Comments

Findings

Figure 2.10.1 Real-time 3D echocardiography (RT3DE). *Left*: four-chamber view showing severe left and right atrial dilation and left ventricular apical involvement. *Right*: longitudinal view, note mitral valve involvement by the disease. Posterior mitral leaflet is involved, showing intense calcification (*arrow*). The anterior mitral leaflet presents a dome-shaped opening.

Figure 2.10.2 RT3DE. Full 3D volume images obtained with angulation. Note a *round* calcification at the apex (*arrows*).

Figure 2.10.3 RT3DE. *Left*: 3D Echo Parametric Imaging derived from the left ventricular 3D volume. *Green* segments contract in a synchronous fashion. Note the presence of late contraction in *red* (*arrows*) that represent the proto-diastolic notch of the interventricular septum, characteristic of a restrictive physiology. *Right*: tissue Doppler imaging at the septum reveals a similar phenomenon (*dashed arrows*).

Case 2.11
■
Tako-Tsubo Syndrome

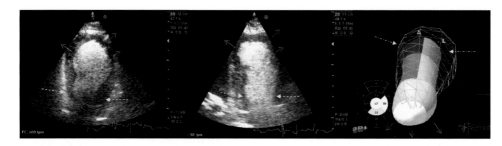

Fig. 2.11.1

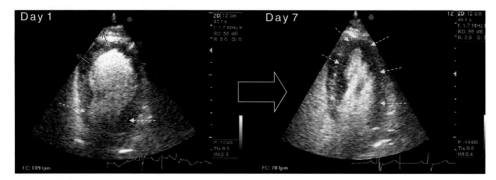

Fig. 2.11.2

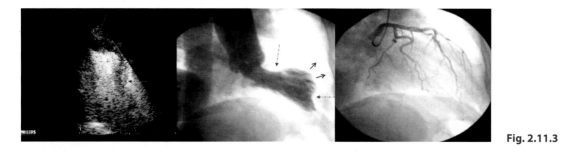

Fig. 2.11.3

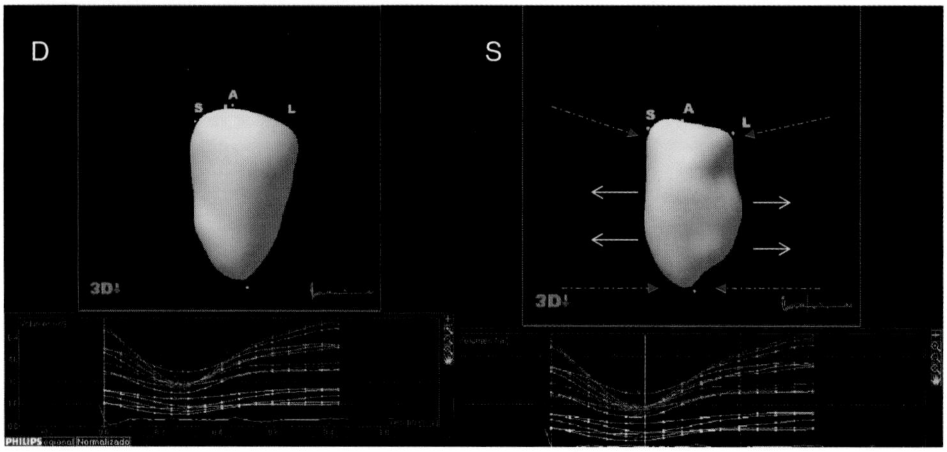

Fig. 2.11.4

We describe cases of two females, 55 and 67 years old, who both presented with prolonged precordial chest pain following deep emotional distress. The younger woman had a strong argument at her job and the older woman recently suffered the death of a beloved relative. Coronary angiogram ruled out obstructive epicardial stenosis in both cases.

The clinical presentation of Tako-Tsubo syndrome (TTS) is similar to that of acute coronary artery syndrome. TTS is far more frequent in females (i.e., 9:1 female/male ratio) and is usually preceded by emotional or physical stress in the absence of epicardial coronary lesions. It is characterized by transient dyskinesia/akinesia, frequently localized in the apex of the left ventricle (LV), although it can affect other areas of the LV such as the mid-ventricular area. In TTS it is common to find ECG abnormalities in the precordial leads and mild troponine elevation. Echocardiography is diagnostic, revealing pathognomonic LV segmental abnormalities in motility as previously described. In addition, echocardiography is essential for clinical follow-up, commonly observing normalization of ventricular segmental motility within 30 days.

Figure 2.10.1 Patient with transitory apical ballooning. *Left*: contrast echocardiography, four-chamber apical view showing mid-apical dyskinesia (*dashed arrows*). Center: same findings observed with two-chamber view. *Right*: real-time 3D echocardiogram (RT3DE), note the segmental abnormalities in 3D LV volume. Dyskinesia of the apical segments (*arrows*) and normal motility at the basal segments (*dashed arrows*).

Figure 2.10.2 *Left*: contrast echocardiography, four-chamber apical view on day 1 showing mid-apical diskenesia. *Right*: similar technique on day 7 showing improvement of apical segmental motility, while LV acquired normal shape.

Figure 2.10.3 Patient with transitory mid-ventricular dyskinesia. *Left*: contrast echocardiography, two-chamber apical view showing antero-medial dyskinesia. *Center*: contrast left ventriculogram during cardiac catheterization showing same echocardiographic findings. *Right*: coronary angiography with no significant left coronary lesions.

Figure 2.10.4 RT3DE, 3D LV volume. *Left*: (diastole) note normal morphology of the left ventricle during diastole. *Right*: (systole) note expansion of mid-ventricular LV (*arrows*) with normal motility at the basal and apical segments (*dashed arrows*).

Case 2.12

Rheumatic Mitral Stenosis

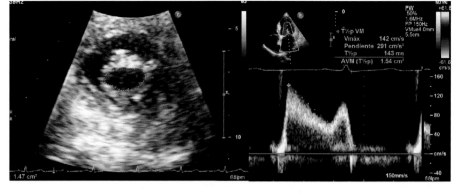

Fig. 2.12.1

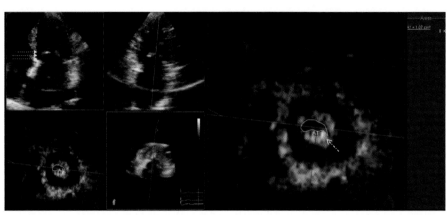

Fig. 2.12.2

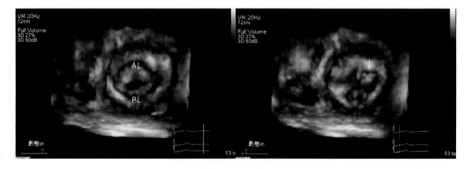

Fig. 2.12.3

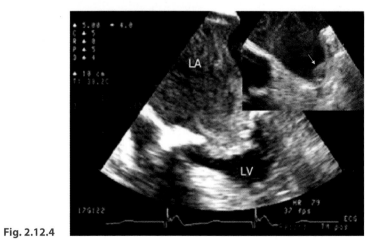

Fig. 2.12.4

A 68-year-old female with surgical commisurotomy 25 years ago was referred for an echocardiogram due to new-onset dyspnea on minimal exertion. An echocardiogram was performed to determine mitral area and select the appropriate therapeutic approach.

Despite reduction in rheumatic fever prevalence, rheumatic mitral stenosis (MS) remains a frequent cause of valvular disease in underdeveloped countries, representing 12% of all valvular cases. 2D and color Doppler echocardiography (2DE) precisely estimate the degree of stenosis and help select the best therapy for MS. Nevertheless, prior surgical procedures in the valve, uncontrolled atrial fibrillation, or concomitant presence of aortic insufficiency limit 2DE conventional assessment (i.e., planimetry, pressure half-time). In these cases, real-time 3D echocardiography (RT3DE) allows a more reliable quantification of MS than 2DE.

The ability to achieve multiple views of the mitral valve in different spatial planes allows adequate alignment with the valve and, hence, precise measurement of the valve area in the most stenotic region.

Furthermore, RT3DE offers detailed anatomical information of the valve and its apparatus, which is very useful to determine feasibility of percutaneous mitral valvuloplasty (PVM) and also guide the procedure. In patients who are candidates for PVM, transesophageal echocardiography (TEE) prior to the procedure is also needed to exclude thrombus in the atriums, which constitutes a contraindication for the percutaneous procedure.

Figure 2.12.1 2DE. *Left*: assessment of mitral valve area by planimetry. *Right*: Doppler tracing assessing pressure half-time. The area by both methods was 1.5 cm². Taking into account that the patient had prior open commisurotomy, the evaluation was further complemented with RT3DE.

Figure 2.12.2 RT3DE. *Left*: assessment of mitral area with multiplanar technique. RT3DE allows transversal view from annulus to the valvular border, until the minimum valvular orifice is encountered. The latter can be achieved without losing proper vertical axis alignment with the heart. *Right*: mitral area was 1.07 (significantly lower than with 2DE).

Figure 2.12.3 RT3DE assessed mitral valve structures. *Left*: (diastole) note considerable thickening of the valve with commissural fusion. *Right*: (systole) nodular calcification is observed at the antero-lateral commissure (*arrow*), which reduces PVM chances of success and increases risk of residual mitral insufficiency. *AL* anterior leaflet; *PL* posterior leaflet.

Figure 2.12.4 TEE: left atrium with severe spontaneous contrast. Zoomed image at the level of the left atrium appendage: note the presence of thrombus (*arrow*), which contraindicates PVM. *LA* left atrium; *LV* left ventricle.

Case 2.13

■

Atrial Septal Defect and Stroke

A 29-year-old female complaining of severe left hemicranial headache, diminished right-eye vision, nausea and vomiting presented to the emergency department. Physical examination revealed right superior quadrantanopsia. Head computed tomography showed occipital attenuation compatible with ischemia at the left posterior cerebral artery. Later on, a magnetic resonance imaging revealed cortical and subcortical edema of the left inferior occipital lobe compatible with a subacute ischemic lesion. ECG was normal. Transthoracic (TTE) and transesophageal echocardiogram (TEE) were done to seek a cardiovascular embolic source.

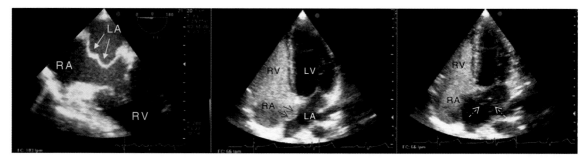

Fig. 2.13.1

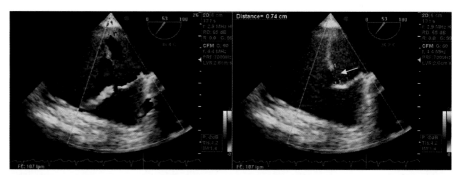

Fig. 2.13.2

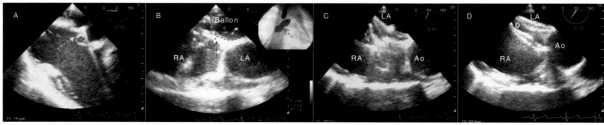

Fig. 2.13.3

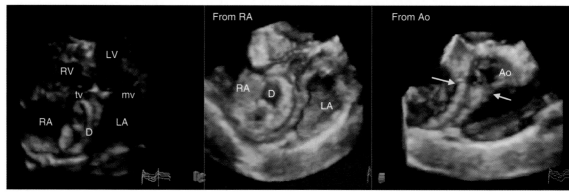

Fig. 2.13.4

Patent foramen ovale (PFO) and atrial septal aneurysm are shown to be at increased risk of ischemic stroke. In young patients with cryptogenic stroke, TTE and TEE are indicated while searching for an embolic source. TTE with agitated saline injection is very sensitive for the detection of PFO and constitutes the first diagnosis step. In this test, correct bubble visualization is performed with harmonic imaging during a Valsalva maneuver. TEE is essential and complementary to TTE, since its use provides detailed information of the atrial septum, which is particularly useful for diagnosis and selection of the best candidates for percutaneous closure. In addition, TEE provides useful guidance during the entire percutaneous procedure (i.e., crossing through the defect, measuring the orifice during balloon inflation, positioning and deployment of the device, assessment of immediate results, and exclusion of potential complications). Nowadays, TEE 3D offers superb anatomical evaluation and may possibly replace bidimensional evaluation in the near future.

Whenever atrial shunt is observed from right to left, the most frequent cause is an association of atrial septal aneurysm and PFO. In rare cases, right to left shunt can be observed in small punctiform atrial septal defects (ostium secundum). In atrial septal defects, the flow is predominantly left to right; thus, the occurrence of cerebrovascular accidents is very low. In the present case, we found a large atrial septal aneurysm with a small septal defect (7 mm) and predominant left to right flow. Nevertheless, in some cardiac beats, the atrial septum presented excursion to the left atrium (LA), detecting a minimal right to left shunt. Based on this observation, we proceeded with percutaneous closure with an Amplatzer device under TEE-guidance. The patient underwent a follow-up TEE 3D.

Figure 2.13.1 TEE. *Right*: conventional mid-esophageal 0° view. Note a large atrial septal aneurysm with a peculiar shape (bilobulated) and excursion to the right atrium (RA, *arrows*). *Center*: Transtoracic echocardiography, 4 chamber view with agitated saline. Note the excursion of the atrial septum to the LA during the relaxation phase, provoked by Valsalva maneuver (*red arrows*). *Left*: Same view by ETT. Note the bubbles passing to the LA (*dashed arrows*).

Figure 2.13.2 TEE. *Left*: color image, 53° view. Note shunt left to right compatible with atrial septal defect, ostium secundum type. *Right*: at the same view without color, note the 7 mm atrial septal defect (*arrow*).

Figure 2.13.3 TEE. Monitoring during percutaneous closure. (a) Threading of the guidewire through the septal defect (*arrow*). (b) Measurement of the defect during balloon inflation. The measurement is taken at the balloon notch (*arrow*). (c) Device with both discs spread out prior to deployment (*arrow*). (d) Assessment after device deployment showing adequate placement, adjacent to the aorta.

Figure 2.13.4 Follow-up evaluation with RT3DE. *Left*: full volume 3D (postprocessed), showing four chambers and their relationship with the device. *Center*: view from RA, showing its relationship with the tricuspid valve. *Right*: view from the aorta, showing the device (*arrow*) properly placed and its relationship with the aorta.

Case 2.14

■

Percutaneous Closure of Severe Paravalvular Leak

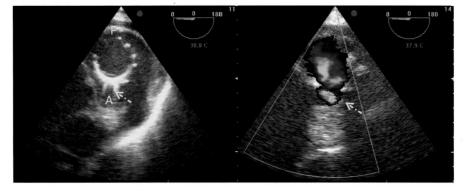

Fig. 2.14.1

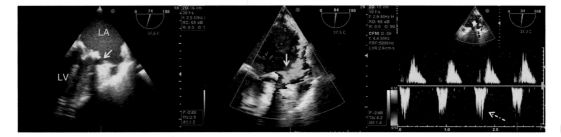

Fig. 2.14.2

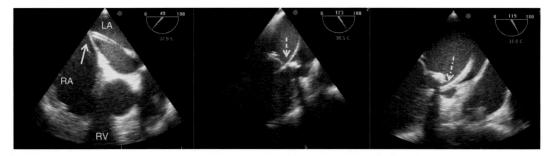

Fig. 2.14.3

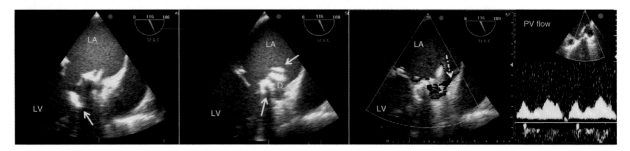

Fig. 2.14.4

An 83-year-old male, former smoker with prior surgical valve replacement (biological prosthesis) due to flail mitral valve 9 years ago, was admitted due to new-onset heart failure. Transesophageal echocardiography (TEE) revealed severe paravalvular leak (PVL) and the possibility of percutaneous closure was considered.

Comments

Reoperation for either replacement or repair of cardiac valve prosthesis is usually recommended in patients with significant PVL. However, in patients unsuitable for cardiac surgery, percutaneous closure of PVL may be considered. Percutaneous closure of PVL is usually performed under general anesthesia, with radiographic and TEE guidance. TEE provides a detailed analysis of the prosthetic dehiscence prior to the intervention, since it evaluates the degree of PVL, the shape and precise location of the dehiscence. During the procedure, TEE guides trans-septal puncture as well as the maneuver and placement of the closing device. Moreover, TEE allows adequate visualization during device deployment and assessment of immediate results (i.e., presence of residual leak). Finally, potential complications such as development of cardiac thrombi, prosthesis regurgitation, or blockade are excluded at the end of the procedure with TEE.

Findings

Figure 2.14.1 TEE. *Left*: conventional 74° view, note PVL on the anterior region (*arrow*), adjacent to the left atrium (LA) appendix. *Center*: color Doppler tracing at 84° view. Note the large periprosthetic regurgitant jet through the dehiscence (*arrow*). *Right*: pulsed Doppler image obtained at the level of the superior left pulmonary vein. Note systolic flow reversal secondary to severe mitral regurgitation (*arrow*). *RA* right atrium.

Figure 2.14.2 TEE. *Left*: conventional transgastric 0° view. *Right*: color Doppler image (systole) at the same level, note the regurgitant orifice at the anterior annular region (*arrow*). *A* anterior; *P* posterior.

Figure 2.14.3 Monitoring percutaneous closure of PVL by TEE (I). *Left*: Conventional, 49° view, showing a correctly localized trans-septal puncture (*arrow*). *Center*: incorrect threading of the guidewire through the valve leaflets (*arrow*). *Right*: correct passage of guidewire and introducer through the dehiscence orifice (*arrow*). *RV* right ventricle.

Figure 2.14.4 TEE. Monitoring percutaneous closure of PVL by TEE (II). *Left*: conventional 116° view, showing deployment of the first device disc at the ventricular side. *Center*: same view after deployment, showing correct placement with no interference in prosthetic valve function. *Right*: color Doppler at the same view, note minimal residual leak (*arrow*). Significant change in pulmonary vein flow pattern is observed with similar systolic and diastolic flow velocities. *LV* left ventricle; *D* device; *PV* pulmonary vein.

Case 2.15
■
Aortic Root Pseudoaneurysm Following Bentall Procedure

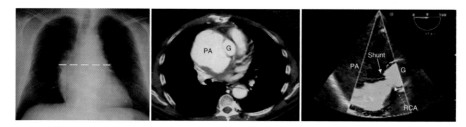

Fig. 2.15.1

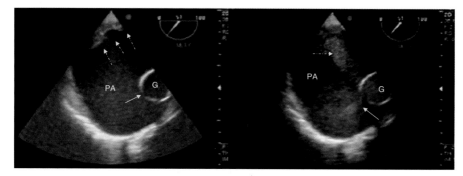

Fig. 2.15.2

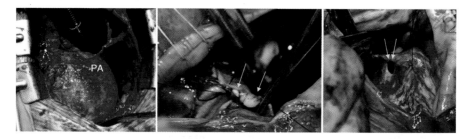

Fig. 2.15.3

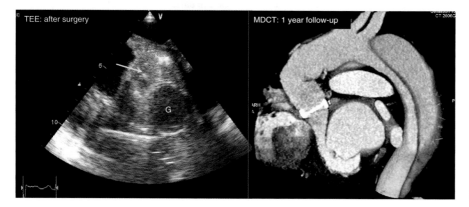

Fig. 2.15.4

We present a case of a 48-year-old hypertensive male with a family history of aortic dissection, and a prior history of aortic dissection type A (aorta 45 mm diameter), associated with moderate to severe aortic valve insufficiency (tricuspid valve) and obstruction of both right and left coronary ostium. The patient underwent a Bentall surgical procedure with concomitant myocardial revascularization (two vein grafts to left and right coronary arteries). Two months later, he returned to our clinic due to new onset of dyspnea and asthenia without signs of heart failure. Hemoglobin level was 9.6 mg/ml, hematocrit 25%. Transesophageal echocardiogram (TEE) and chest computed tomography were done.

Comments

The incidence of pseudoaneurysm formation unrelated to infection in patients who have undergone aortic root replacement (Bentall procedure) is at least 8–10%.

The communication point is more commonly situated at the suture of the right coronary ostium; however, communications may exist distal to the suture or fistulas to right atrium. Pseudoaneurysm formation can occur over variable lengths of time. Immediate postoperative and follow-up assessment by imaging techniques contributes to an early diagnosis and treatment of this complication. By providing substantial morphological and functional data, TEE remains superior to transthoracic (TTE) for the diagnosis of this complex complication. In addition, TEE conveys information regarding the communication points between the prosthetic tube and the pseudoaneurysm. Furthermore, TEE with contrast administration unmasked discrete communication points not diagnosed by other imaging techniques. The latter is vital prior to reoperation. Multislice computed tomography (MSCT) offers more detailed information with greater vision perspective. In many cases, multiple imaging techniques are necessary in order to perform a precise diagnosis and select the best surgical strategy.

Findings

Figure 2.15.1 *Left*: chest-X-ray during readmission to the hospital revealing a widened mediastinum. *Center*: Helicoidal CT demonstrating a cavity adjacent to the aorta with mural thrombus compatible with pseudoaneurysm (PA) formation. *Right*: color TEE at mid-esophageal 0° view. Note the jet from the graft to the pseudoaneurysm at the level of the proximal anastomosis of the vein grafted to right coronary artery (*arrow*).

Figure 2.15.2 TEE. *Left*: conventional image at mid-esophageal 0° view, note a large pseudoaneurysm with mural thrombus (*dashed arrows*). Note complete tear of the proximal anastomosis to right coronary artery (*arrow*). *Right*: contrast image at the same view, revealing the presence of two jets. One jet communicates the graft to pulmonary artery through the tear of the proximal anastomosis of the vein graft (*arrow*), while a second jet communicates the graft to the right atrium (*dashed arrow*). The start point of the jet is not visualized at the origin in this image.

Figure 2.15.3 Images during surgery. *Left*: external view of the pseudoaneurysm. *Center*: Suture of the vein graft tear to right coronary artery (*arrows*). *Left*: Communication orifice to right atrium (*arrow*).

Figure 2.15.4 *Left*: postoperative TEE at day 1. Note a hematoma adjacent to the tube without internal flow (*arrow*). *Right*: MSCT. Follow-up after 1 year, showing resolution of pseudoaneurysm.

Further Reading

Books

Textbook of Clinical Echocardiography, 3rd ed. Catherine M. Otto (2004) Saunders, Philadelphia

Feigenbaum's Echocardiography. Harvey Feigenbaum, William Armstrong (2004) Lippincott Williams & Wilkins, Philadelphia

The Echo Manual. Jae K. Oh, James B. Seward (2006) Lippincott Williams & Wilkins, Philadelphia

Atlas of Transesophageal Echocardiography. Navin C. Nanda, Michael J. Domanski (2006) Lippincott Williams & Wilkins, Philadelphia

Doppler Myocardial Imaging. A Textbook. George.R Sutherland, Liv Hatle, Piet Claus Jan D' hooge, Bart Bijnens (2006) BSWK, Belgium

Atlas of Intraoperative Transesophageal Echocardiography: Surgical and Radiologic Correlations, Textbook with DVD. Donald Oxorn; Catherine M. Otto (2007) Saunders, Philadelphia

3-D Echocardiography, An Issue of Cardiology Clinics. Edward A. Gill, N. Nanda (2007) Saunders, Philadelphia

López de Sá E, López-Sendón JL, Rubio R. Infarto agudo de miocardio: clínica, evolución y complicaciones. In: Delcán JL (ed) Cardiopatía isquémica. ENE ediciones, Madrid, 1999; 583–584

Rotura Cardiaca Isquémica. Text book. Figueras J, Soler Soler J (2001) Editorial, Doyma

Sbar S, Harrison EE. Chronic tricuspid insufficiency due to trauma. In: Hurst JW (ed) The Heart: Update III. McGraw-Hill, New York, 1980; 43–51

Interactive CD of Echocardiography

Clinical Echocardiography. Arturo Evangelista, Herminio Garcia del Castillo. Co-authors: Teresa Gonzalez Alujas, Gustavo Avegliano, Zamira Bosch. The Academy of Medical Ultrasound. Supported by GE Healthcare, 2004

Web-Links

http://www.wiley.com/bw/journal.asp?ref=0742–2822

http://www.med.yale.edu/intmed/cardio/echo_atlas/contents/index.html

http://asecho.org/

http://journals.elsevierhealth.com/periodicals/ymje

http://www.interscience.wiley.com/jpages/0742–2822

http://www.sciencedirect.com/science/journal/08947317

http://www.escardio.org

Articles

Abad C. Tumores cardiacos (II). Tumores primitivos malignos. Tumores metastásicos. Tumor carcinoide. Rev Esp Cardiol 1998; 51:103–114

Abinder E, Sharif D, Shefer A et al Novel insights into the natural history of apical hypetrophic cardiomyopathy during long-term follow-up. IMAJ 2002; 4:166–169

Acebo E, Val-Bernal JF, Gómez Román JJ. Thrombomodulin, cal-retinin and c-kit (CD117) expression in cardiac myxoma. Histol Histopathol 2001; 16:1031–1036

Ako J. Apical and midventricular transient left ventricular dysfunction syndrome (tako-tsubo cardiomyopathy). Chest 2008; 133(4):1052; author reply 1053

Alcalai R, Seidman J, Seidman C et al Genetic basis of hypertrophic cardiomyopathy: from bench to the clinics J Cardiovasc Electrophysiol 2008; 19:104–110

Almendro-Delia M, Hidalgo-Urbano R. Transient midventricular dyskinesia: tako-tsubo cardiomyopathy. The story continues. Rev Esp Cardiol 2008; 61(11):1223–1224

Aoyagi S, Kosuga K, Akashi H, Oryoji A, Oishi K. Aortic root replacement with a composite graft: results of 69 operations in 66 patients. Ann Thorac Surg 1994; 58:1469–1475

Armstrong WF, Bach DS, Carey LM, Froehlich J, Lowell M, Kazerooni EA. Clinical and echocardiographic findings in patients with suspected acute aortic dissection. Am Heart J 1998; 136:1051–1060

Avegliano G, Evangelista A, Elorz C, González-Alujas T, García del Castillo H, Soler-Soler J. Acute peripheral arterial ischemia and suspected aortic dissection: usefulness of transesophageal echocardiography in differential diagnosis with aortic thrombosis. Am J Cardiol 2002; 90(6):674–677

Belghiti H, Aouad A, Arharbi M. Suspected left-ventricular non-compaction on two- and three-dimensional echocardiography: is it always clear? Arch Card Dis 2008; 101:373–374

Berensztein CS, Piñeiro D, Marcotegui M, Brunoldi R, Blanco MV, Lerman J. Usefulness of echocardiography and Doppler echocardiography in endomyocardial fibrosis. J Am Soc Echocardiogr 2000; 13(5):385–392

Bicudo LS, Tsutsui JM, Shiozaki A et al Value of real time three-dimensional echocardiography in patients with hypertrophic cardiomyopathy: comparison with two-dimensional echocardiography and magnetic resonance imaging. Echocardiography 2008; 25:717–726

Biorck G, Mogensen L, Nyquist O, Orinius E, Sjogren A. Studies of myocardial rupture with tamponade in acute myocardial infarction: clinical features. Chest 1972; 61:4–6

Blockmans D, Bley T, Schmidt W. Imaging for large-vessel vasculitis. Curr Opin Rheumatol 2009; 21(1):19–28

Both M, Ahmadi-Simab K, Reuter M, Dourvos O, Fritzer E, Ullrich S, Gross WL, Heller M, Bähre M. MRI and FDG-PET in the assessment of inflammatory aortic arch syndrome in complicated courses of giant cell arteritis. Ann Rheum Dis 2008; 67(7):1030–1033

Botto F, Trivi M, Padilla LT. Transient left midventricular ballooning without apical involvement. Int J Cardiol 2008; 127(3):e158–e159

Breithardt OA, Becker M, Kälsch T, Haghi D. Follow-up in Tako-tsubo cardiomyopathy by real-time three-dimensional echocardiography. Heart 2008; 94(2):210

Brian C, Weiford MD, Vijay D, Subbarao MD, Kevin M, Mulhern MD. Noncompaction of the ventricular myocardium. Circulation 2004; 109:2965–2971

Bizzarri F, Mattia C, Ricci M, Coluzzi F, Petrozza V, Frati G, Pugliese G, Muzzi L. Cardiogenic shock as a complication of acute mitral valve regurgitation following posteromedial papillary muscle infarction in the absence of coronary artery disease. J Cardiothorac Surg 2008; 3:61

Cellarier G, Cuguillière A, Gisserot O, Laurent P, Bouchiat C, Bonal J, Talard P, Dussarat GV. Acute complication of a composite graft replacement of the aortic root. J Mal Vasc 1999; 24(5):381–383

Chan KL. Usefulness of transesophageal echocardiography in the diagnosis of conditions mimicking aortic dissection. Am Heart J 1991; 122:495–504

Chin TK, Perloff JK, Williams RG et al Isolated noncompaction of left ventricular myocardium: a study of eight cases. Circulation 1990; 82:507–513

Chirillo F et al Usefulness of transthoracic and transoesophageal echocardiography in recognition and management of cardiovascular injuries after blunt chest trauma. Heart 1996; 75(3):301–306

Costabel JP, Avegliano G et al Miocardiopatía hipertrófica apical que simula um síndrome coronario agudo. Utilidad de la ecocardiografía tridimensional. Rev Argent Cardiol 2008; 76:488–490 (spanish text)

Daniel WG, Nellessen U, Schröder E, Nonnast-Daniel B, Bednarski P, Nikutta P, Lichtlen PR. Left atrial spontaneous echo contrast in mitral valve disease: an indicator for an increased thromboembolic risk. J Am Coll Cardiol 1988; 11(6):1204–1211

DeBakey ME, McCollum CH, Crawford ES. Dissection and dissecting aneurysms of the aorta: twenty-year follow-up of five hundred twenty-seven patients treated surgically. Surgery 1982; 92:1118–1134

Delgado Ramis L, Montiel J, Arís A, Caralps JM. Rotura traumática de la válvula tricúspide: presentación de tres casos. Rev Esp Cardiol 2000; 53:874–877

Eliot RS, Baroldi G, Leone A. Necropsy studies in myocardial infarction with minimal or no coronary luminal reduction due to atherosclerosis. Circulation 1974; 49(6):1127–1131

Erbel R, Börner N, Bruñiré J et al Detection of aortic dissection by transoesophageal echocardiography. Br Heart J 1987; 58: 45–51

Ericsson M, Sonnenberg B, Woo A et al Long-term outcome in patients with apical hypertrophic cardiomyopathy. J Am Coll Cardiol 2002; 39(4):638–645

Evangelista A. Puesta al día en el diagnóstico y tratamiento del sindróme aórtico agudo. Rev Esp Cardiol 2007; 60(4):428–439

Evangelista A, González Alujas T, Garcia del Castillo H et al Ecocardiografía transesofágica en el diagnóstico de la disección aórtica. Rev Esp Cardiol 1993; 46:805–809

Fabricius AM, Walther T, Falk V, Mohr FW. Three-dimensional echocardiography for planning of mitral valve surgery: current applicability?Ann Thorac Surg 2004; 78(2):575–578

Figueras J, Alcalde O, Barrabés JA, Serra V, Alguersuari J, Cortadellas J, Lidón RM. Changes in hospital mortality rates in 425 patients with acute ST-elevation myocardial infarction and cardiac rupture over a 30-year period. Circulation 2008; 118(25):2783–2789

Figueras J, Cortadellas J, Calvo F, Soler-Soler J. Relevance of delayed hospital admission on development of cardiac rupture during acute myocardial infarction: study in 225 patients with free wall, septal or papillary muscle rupture. J Am Coll Cardiol 1998; 32:135–139

Frans E, Nanda N, Patel V et al Live three dimensional transthoracic contrast echocardiographic assessment of apical cardiomyopathy. Ecocardiology 2005; 22(8)686–689

Gayet C, Pierre B, Delahaye J, Champsaur G, Andre-Fouet X, Rueff P. Traumatic tricuspid insufficiency, an underdiagnosed disease. Chest 1987; 92:429–432

Gopalamurugan AB, Kapetanakis S, Monaghan M. Left ventricular non-compaction diagnosed by real time three dimensional echocardiography. Heart 2005; 10:1274

Gutiérrez-Chico JL, Zamorano Gómez JL, Rodrigo-López JL, Mataix L, Pérez de Isla L, Almería-Valera C, Aubele A, Macaya-Miguel C. Accuracy of real-time 3-dimensional echocardiog-

raphy in the assessment of mitral prolapse. Is transesophageal echocardiography still mandatory? Am Heart J 2008; 155(4): 694–698

Haddad M, Veinot JP, Masters RG, Hendry PJ. Essential thrombocytosis causing a massive myocardial infarction. Cardiovasc Pathol 2003; 12(4):216–218

Hagan PG, Nienaber CA, Isselbacher EM, Bruckman D, Karavite DJ, Russman PL, Evangelista A. The international registry of acute aortic dissection (IRAD). New insights into an old disease. JAMA 2000; 283:897–903

Hirata K, Pulerwitz T, Sciacca R, Otsuka R, Oe Y, Fujikura K, Oe H, Hozumi T, Yoshiyama M, Yoshikawa J, Di Tullio M, Homma S. Clinical utility of new real time three-dimensional transthoracic echocardiography in assessment of mitral valve prolapse. Echocardiography 2008; 25(5):482–488

Hozumi T, Yoshikawa J, Yoshida K, Akasaka T, Takagi T, Yamamuro A. Assessment of flail mitral leaflets by dynamic three-dimensional echocardiographic imaging. Am J Cardiol 1997; 79(2): 223–225

Hutt MS. Epidemiology aspects of endomyocardial fibrosis. Postgrad Med J 1983; 59(689):142–146

Illarroel MT et al Traumatic tricuspid insufficiency. Rev Esp Cardiol 1989; 42(2):145–147

Jenni R, Oechslin E, Schneider J, Attenhofer Jost C, Kaufmann PA. Echocardiographic and pathoanatomical characteristics of isolated left ventricular non-compaction: a step towards classification as a distinct cardiomyopathy. Heart 2001; 86(6): 666–671

Jenni R, Oechslin EN, van der Loo B. Isolated ventricular non-compaction of the myocardium in adults. Heart 2007; 93(1): 11–15

Kitaoka H, Doi Y, Casey S, Hitomi N et al Comparison of prevalence of apical hypertrophic cardiomyopathy in Japan and the United States. Am J Cardiol 2003; 92(10):1183–1186

Koo BK, Choi D, Ha J et al Isolated noncompaction of the ventricular myocardium: contrast echocardiographic findings and review of the literature. Echocardiography 2002; 19:153–156

Kouchoukos NT, Wareing TH, Murphy SF, Perrillo JB. Sixteen-year experience with aortic root replacement. Results of 172 operations. Ann Surg 1991; 214:308–320

Kuppahally SS, Paloma A, Craig Miller D, Schnittger I, Liang D. Multiplanar visualization in 3D transthoracic echocardiography for precise delineation of mitral valve pathology. Echocardiography 2008; 25(1):84–87

Kühl HP, Hoffmann R, Merx MW, Franke A, Klötzsch C, Lepper W, Reineke T, Noth J, Hanrath P. Transthoracic echocardiography using second harmonic imaging: diagnostic alternative to transesophageal echocardiography for the detection of atrial right to left shunt in patients with cerebral embolic events. J Am Coll Cardiol 1999; 34(6):1823–1830

Laraudogoitia E, Evangelista A, Garci'a del Castillo H, Lekuona I, Palomar S, González Alujas T, Salcedo A. Thombus of the thoracic aorta as a source of peripheral embolism diagnosed by transesophageal echocardiography. Rev EspCardiol 1997; 50:62–64

Laperche T, Laurian C, Roudaut R, Steg G. Mobile thromboses of the aortic arch without aortic debris. A transesophageal echocardiographic finding associated with unexplained arterial embolism. Circulation 1997; 96:288–294

López-Sendón J, González A, López de Sá E, Coma-Canella I, Roldán I, Domínguez F et al Diagnosis of subacute ventricular wall rupture after acute myocardial infarction: sensitivity and specificity of clinical, hemodynamic and echocardiographic criteria. J Am Coll Cardiol 1992; 19:1145–1153

Mattioli AV, Aquilina M, Oldani A, Longhini C, Mattioli G. Atrial septal aneurysm as a cardioembolic source in adult patients with stroke and normal carotid arteries. A multicentre study. Eur Heart J 2001; 22(3):261–268

Messika-Zeitoun D, Brochet E, Holmin C, Rosenbaum D, Cormier B, Serfaty JM, Iung B, Vahanian A. Three-dimensional evaluation of the mitral valve area and commissural opening before and after percutaneous mitral commissurotomy in patients with mitral stenosis. Eur Heart J 2007; 28(1):72–79

Miller DC, Mitchell RS, Oyer PE, Stinson EB, Jamieson SW, Shumway NE. Independent determinants of operative mortality for patients with aortic dissections. Circulation 1984; 70(suppl I):I-153–I-164

Moon J, Fisher N, McKenna W et al Detection of apical hypertrophic cardiomyopathy by cardiovascular magnetic resonance in patients with non-diagnostic echocardiography. Heart 2007; 90(6)645–649

Moukarbel G, Alam S, Abchee A. Contrast-enhanced echocardiography for the diagnosis of apical hypertrophic cardiomyopathy. Echocardiography 2005; 22:831–833

Müller S, Müller L, Laufer G, Alber H, Dichtl W, Frick M, Pachinger O, Bartel T. Comparison of three-dimensional imaging to transesophageal echocardiography for preoperative evaluation in mitral valve prolapse. Am J Cardiol 2006; 98(2): 243–248

Naja I, Barriuso C, Ninot S, Martínez C, Oller G, Nolla M et al Rotura traumática de la válvula tricúspide. Tratamiento quirúrgico conservador. Rev Esp Cardiol 1992; 45:64–66

Oechslin E, Jenni R. Isolated left ventricular non-compaction: increasing recognition of this distinct, yet 'unclassified' cardiomyopathy. Eur J Echocardiogr 2002; 3(4):250–251

Omeroglu SN, Mansuroglu D, Goksedef D, Cevat Y. Ultrafast computed tomography in management of post-bentall aortic root pseudoaneurysm repair. Tex Heart Inst J 2005; 32(1): 91–94

Oliva PO, Hammill SC, Edwards WE. Cardiac rupture, a clinically predictable complication of acute myo-cardial infarction: report of 70 cases with clinicopathologic correlations. J Am Coll Cardiol 1993; 22:720–726

Orihashi K, Sueda T, Okada K, Imai K. Perioperative diagnosis of mesenteric ischemia in acute aortic dissection by transesophageal echocardiography. Eur J Cardiothorac Surg 2005; 28(6): 871–876

Pacifico L, Spodick D. ILEAD-ischemia of the lower extremities due to aortic dissection: the isolated presentation. Clin Cardiol 1999; 22:353–356

Pappas PJ, Cernainau AC, Baldino WA, Cilley JH Jr, Del Rossi AJ. Ventricular free wall rupture after myocardial infarction: treatment and outcome. Chest 1991; 99:892–895

Patel AK, D'Arbela PG, Somers K. Endomyocardial fibrosis and eosinophilia. Br Heart J 1977; 39(3):238–241

Patel KC, Pennell D, Leyva-Leon F. Left ventricular trabecular non-compaction. Heart 2004; 90(9):1076

Perez de Isla L, Casanova C, Almería C, Rodrigo JL, Cordeiro P, Mataix L, Aubele AL, Lang R, Zamorano JL. Which method should be the reference method to evaluate the severity of rheumatic mitral stenosis? Gorlin's method versus 3D-echo. Eur J Echocardiogr 2007; 8(6):470–473

Pepi M, Tamborini G, Maltagliati A, Galli CA, Sisillo E, Salvi L, Naliato M, Porqueddu M, Parolari A, Zanobini M, Alamanni F.

Head-to-head comparison of two- and three-dimensional transthoracic and transesophageal echocardiography in the localization of mitral valve prolapse. J Am Coll Cardiol 2006; 48(12):2524–2530

Petersen SE, Selvanayagam JB, Wiesmann F, Robson MD, Francis JM, Anderson RH, Watkins H, Neubauer S. Left ventricular non-compaction: insights from cardiovascular magnetic resonance imaging. J Am Coll Cardiol. 2005 5;46(1):101–5

Pinar Sopena J, Candell Riera J, San José Laporte A, Bosch Gil J, García del Castillo H, Vilardell Tarres M, Soler Soler J. Echocardiographic manifestations in patients with hypereosinophilia. Rev Esp Cardiol 1990; 43(7):450–456 (Spanish)

Pothineni KR, Duncan K, Yelamanchili P, Nanda NC et al Live/real time three-dimensional transthoracic echocardiographic assessment of tricuspid valve pathology: incremental value over the two-dimensional technique. Echocardiography 2007; 24(5): 541–552

Prichard RW. Tumors of the heart: review of the subject and report of one hundred and fifty cases. Arch Patol 1951; 51: 98–128

Ramphal PS, Spencer HW, Mitchell DI. Myxoma of right femoralvein origin presenting as right atrial mass with syncope. J Thorac Cardiovasc Surg 1998; 116:655–656

Reddy VK, Nanda S, Bandarupalli N, Pothineni KR, Nanda NC. Traumatic tricuspid papillary muscle and chordae rupture: emerging role of three-dimensional echocardiography. Echocardiography 2008; 25(6):653–657

Reynen K. Cardiac myxomas. N Engl J Med 1995; 333: 1610–1617

Reyen K. Frequency of primary tumors of the heart. Am J Cardiol 1996; 77:107

Roberts WC. Primary and secondary neoplasms of the heart. Am J Cardiol 1997; 80:671–682

Russo A, Suri RM, Grigioni F, Roger VL, Oh JK, Mahoney DW, Schaff HV, Enriquez-Sarano M. Clinical outcome after surgical correction of mitral regurgitation due to papillary muscle rupture. Circulation 2008; 118(15):1528–1534

Saffitz JE, Phillips ER, Temesy-Armos PN, Roberts WC. Thrombocytosis and fatal coronary heart disease. Am J Cardiol 1983; 52(5):651–652

Seelos KC, Funari M, Higgins CB. Detection of aortic arch thrombus using MR imaging. J Comput Assist Tomogr 1991; 15:244–247

Sharma R, Mann J, Drummond L, Livesey SA, Simpson IA. The evaluation of real-time 3-dimensional transthoracic echocardiography for the preoperative functional assessment of patients with mitral valve prolapse: a comparison with 2-dimensional transesophageal echocardiography. J Am Soc Echocardiogr 2007; 20(8):934–940

Soyer H, Laudinat JM, Lemaitre C, Pommier JL, Delepine G, Poncet A, Baehrel B, Bajolet A. Recurrent mobile thrombus of the ascending aorta diagnosed by transesophageal echocardiography. Arch Mal Coeur 1993; 86:1769–1771

Spry CJ, Take M, Tai PC. Eosinophilic disorders affecting the myocardium and endocardium: a review. Heart Vessels Suppl 1985; 1:240–242

Suzuki T, Metha R, Ince H, Nagai R, Sakomura Y, Weber F. Clinical profiles and outcomes of acute type B aortic dissection in the current era: lessons from the International Registry of Aortic Dissection (IRAD). Circulation 2003; 108(suppl II): II-312–II-317

Szczytowski JM, Mixon TA, Santos RA, Lawrence ME. Images in cardiovascular medicine. A 54-year-old woman with chest pain, dyspnea, and inferior injury on electrocardiography. Circulation 2006; 113(23):e852

Terracciano LM, Mhawech P, Suess K, D'Armiento M, Lehmann FS, Jundt G et al Calretinin as a marker for cardiac myxoma. Diagnostic and histogenetic considerations. Am J Clin Pathol 2000; 114:754–759

Van Son J, Danielson G, Schaff H, Miller F. Traumatic tricuspid valve insufficiency. J Thorac Cardiovasc Surg 1994; 108: 893–898

Varnava AM. Isolated left ventricular non-compaction: a distinct cardiomyopathy? Heart 2001; 86(6):599–600

Virmani R, Popovsky MA, Roberts WC. Thrombocytosis, coronary thrombosis and acute myocardial infarction. Am J Med 1979; 67(3):498–506

Vitebskiy S, Fox K, Hoit BD. Routine transesophageal echocardiography for the evaluation of cerebral emboli in elderly patients. Echocardiography 2005; 22(9):770–774

Wells KE, Alexander JJ, Piotrowski JJ, Finkelhor RS. Massive aortic thrombus det ected by transesophageal echocardiography as a cause of peripheral emboli in young patients. Am Heart J 1996; 132:882–883

Young JR, Kramer J, Humphries AW. The ischemic leg: a clue to dissecting aneurysm. Cardiovasc Clin 1975; 7:201–205

Zamorano J, Cordeiro P, Sugeng L, Perez de Isla L, Weinert L, Macaya C, Rodríguez E, Lang RM. Real-time three-dimensional echocardiography for rheumatic mitral valve stenosis evaluation: an accurate and novel approach. J Am Coll Cardiol 2004; 43(11):2091–2096

Zamorano J, Perez de Isla L, Sugeng L, Cordeiro P, Rodrigo JL, Almeria C, Weinert L, Feldman T, Macaya C, Lang RM, Hernandez Antolin R. Non-invasive assessment of mitral valve area during percutaneous balloon mitral valvuloplasty: role of real-time 3D echocardiography. Eur Heart J 2004; 25(23):2086–2091

Cardiac Magnetic Resonance

Joan C. Vilanova, Antonio Luna, Manel Morales, Xavier Albert, Joaquim Barceló, and Ramón Ribes

Introduction

Cardiovascular magnetic resonance has emerged as an important clinical tool in the last decade. Technical advances in cardiothoracic MR imaging have expanded from a primary tomographic imaging modality to a dynamic one. Today it is possible to acquire high-resolution imaging of ventricular function, valvular motion, and myocardial perfusion. In addition, cardiac MRI is now considered the "gold standard" for the assessment of regional and global ventricular function, myocardial infarction, delayed enchancement, and congenital heart disease.

Cardiac MR offers several advantages over other diagnostic imaging methods. First, it does not use ionizing radiation. Second, it provides additional diagnostic information about tissue characteristics. Finally, MRI provides three-dimensional (3D) images many desired plane.

In the past, cardiac MR was primarily a research tool, and scans for clinical purposes were rare and performed primarily for pathologies such as arrhythmogenic right ventricular cardiomyopathy and cardiac neoplasms.

CMR is considered a complementary study to echocardiography, as it is still the first choice for the diagnosis and follow-up of multiple cardiac diseases when the latter is inconclusive for a specific cardiac pathology or due to technical difficulties. Since the introduction of CMR in daily clinical practice, the number of clinical situations in which CMR is indicated has continued to grow.

Despite the progression of CMR, general acceptance has progressed slowly. Although multifactorial, this slow acceptance is primarily due to two reasons. First, referring physicians remain unfamiliar with the wide variety of CMR examinations that are available for routine clinical use, and second, clinical expertise in the practice of CMR is scarce and limited to few centers. The expanding availability of cardiac MR education will likely alleviate these bottlenecks.

During the past years, as cardiac MR imaging has become more common and image quality has improved, increasing recognition of the power of this imaging methods for the investigation of cardiac disease has stimulated great interest in the radiology community.

The recent developments in MR imaging provide shorter imaging times and improved resolution, resulting in improved tissue characterization and enhanced diagnostic accuracy.

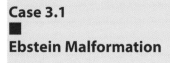

Case 3.1
■
Ebstein Malformation

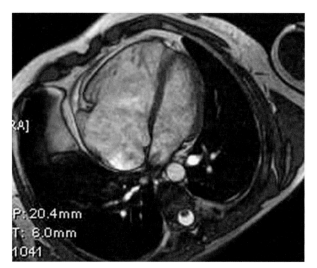

Fig. 3.1.1

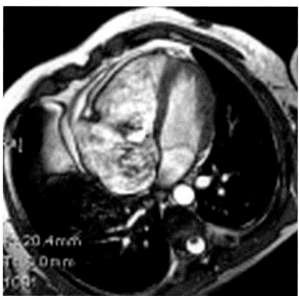

Fig. 3.1.2

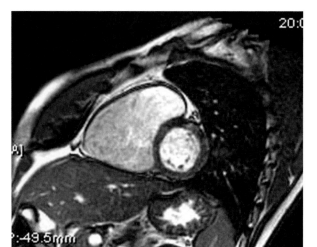

Fig. 3.1.3

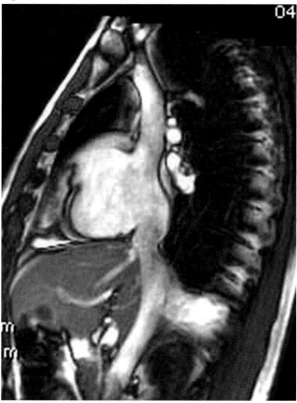

Fig. 3.1.4

An obese 26-year-old male patient with no toxic habits or relevant history apart from a heart murmur discovered during childhood and never studied consulted a general practitioner for dyspnea on exertion and brief, isolated episodes of palpitations. Chest X-ray showed cardiomegaly affecting the right chambers, with no signs of left heart failure. The EKG showed sinus rhythm with complete right branch block. The patient was referred to a cardiologist, who performed echocardiography and found dilated right chambers and severe tricuspid regurgitation and requested a cardiac MRI examination.

Introduction

Cardiac MRI is very useful for the study of the right ventricle, which can at times be limited in the echocardiogram. In this patient, in addition to the right chambers, we studied the venous drainage from both atria and found it correct without shunts. The interventricular and interatrial septa were intact. Atrialization of the right ventricle compatible with Ebstein malformation and severe tricuspid regurgitation was observed. A common finding in this congenital anomaly is abnormal attachments of the tricuspid valve leaflets, with displacement of the septal and posterior leaflets into the cavity of the right ventricle. As a consequence, severe tricuspid regurgitation can occur and cause dilatation of both the right ventricle and the right atrium. This anomaly may be associated to coarctation of the aorta, alterations in the mitral valve, right outflow tract obstruction, interventricular shunts, or patent ductus arteriosus. These alterations were ruled out during the examination.

Indications for surgical correction of Ebstein malformation include substantial cyanosis, right heart failure, very limited functional capacity (NYHA class III), and possibly the recurrence of paradoxical emboli (50% of these patients have a permeable foramen ovale). Relative indications include arrhythmias that cannot be controlled with medication or ablation and a cardiothoracic index greater than 65% in asymptomatic patients.

Cardiac MRI Findings

End-diastolic 4-chamber view bright-blood steady-state free-precession (SSFP-FIESTA) image shows significant dilatation of the right chambers with high implantation of the septal leaflet of the tricuspid valve with respect to the mitral plane that reaches 20 mm in the four-chamber view (Fig. 3.1.1). End-systolic 4-chamber view SSFP-FIESTA cine image shows the significant turbulence at the level of the right atrium, compatible with severe tricuspid regurgitation (Fig. 3.1.2). The short-axis view shows the dilatation of the right ventricle in comparison with the left ventricle (Fig. 3.1.3). Two-right-chamber view SSFP-FIESTA cine image including the venae cavae shows the correct drainage of these two veins as well as significant dilatation of the right atrium (Fig. 3.1.4).

Case 3.2
■
Ablation for Ventricular Tachycardia

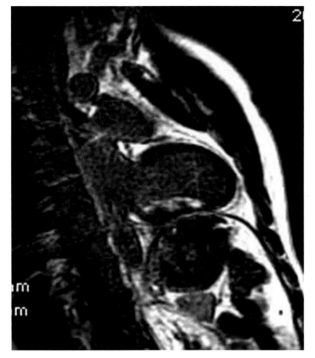

Fig. 3.2.1

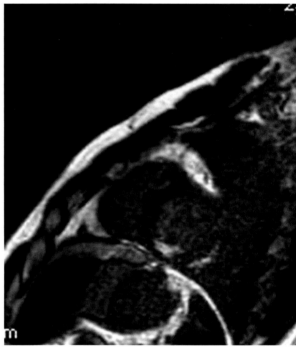

Fig. 3.2.2

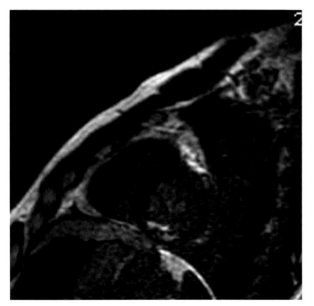

Fig. 3.2.3

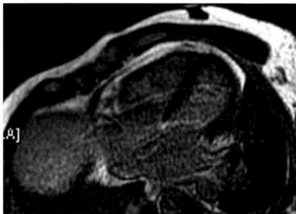

Fig. 3.2.4

A 36-year-old female patient with no toxic habits or relevant history presented with very fast palpitations lasting approximately 5 min, associated to lightheadedness but without chest pain or other symptoms. No alterations were observed on the EKG, electrocardiography, or 24-h Holter. During one episode, the patient presented at the emergency department and the EKG registered wide QRS tachycardia of 220 beats per minute compatible with ventricular tachycardia with right bundle branch block. The patient was admitted for further study.

Another echocardiogram and gadolinium-enhanced cardiac MRI to study the causes of the ventricular tachycardia yielded normal findings. Cardiac catheterization showed normal coronary arteries. Thus, we were faced with idiopathic ventricular tachycardia in a patient with a structurally normal heart who had a normal surface EKG and no significant coronary disease or family history of arrhythmia or sudden death. These ventricular tachycardias are reentry phenomena that originate in the His-Purkinje system in the left heart, giving rise to fascicular tachycardia. When incessant, this type of ventricular tachycardia can lead to tachycardia-induced cardiomyopathy. However, in this case, ventricular function was strictly normal. This type of ventricular tachycardias can be treated by radiofrequency catheter ablation. Although this is a complex ablation procedure, it can cure the patient. In this patient, an electrophysiological study was able to induce the tachycardia so it could be ablated. After ablation, the arrhythmia could not be induced. The patient became asymptomatic and gadolinium-enhanced cardiac MRI perfectly depicted the area of ablation in the inferior mediobasal and posterior mediobasal segments, corresponding to approximately 50% of the thickness of the myocardium. Contractility in these segments was strictly normal on cine MRI sequences.

Long-axis and short-axis views 3D GRE delayed enhancement sequences clearly show the marked contrast uptake at the level of the inferior and posterior mediobasal segments (Figs 3.2.1–3.2.3). In the four-chamber view GRE delayed enhancement sequence no contrast enhancement is evident at the level of the apex, lateral walls, or posterior septum (Fig. 3.2.4).

Case 3.3
■
Dilated Cardiomyopathy

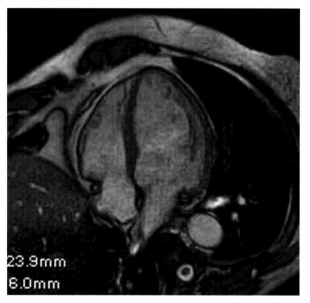

Fig. 3.3.1

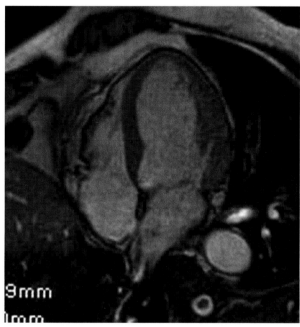

Fig. 3.3.2

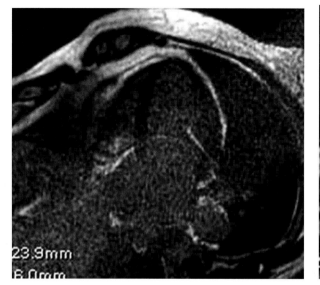

Fig. 3.3.3

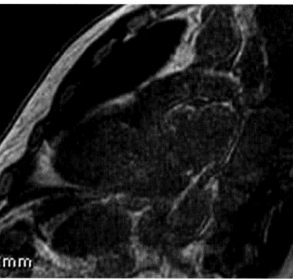

Fig. 3.3.4

A 68-year-old male smoker with type II diabetes mellitus and a history of cholecystectomy for biliary lithiasis 20 years prior presented with shortness of breath of several months' evolution leading to NYHA functional class III with orthopnea and a few episodes of paroxysmal nocturnal dyspnea. The surface EKG showed complete left bundle branch block of the bundle of His. Findings at echocardiography were compatible with dilated cardiomyopathy, with global contractility of the left ventricle affected and a severely depressed ejection fraction of 30% without clear segmental alterations.

Introduction

Before dilated cardiomyopathy can be diagnosed and characterized as idiopathic, the differential diagnosis with dilated cardiomyopathy of ischemic origin must be performed, as the therapeutic approach to these two entities is completely different. Cardiac MRI is very useful in this differential diagnosis, but it cannot replace coronary angiography at this stage. Moreover, cardiac MRI enables us to calculate the ventricular volumes and ejection fractions of both ventricles with great precision and reproducibility, so it is very useful for follow-up. In idiopathic dilated cardiomyopathy, systolic dysfunction is usually diffuse and there is a greater degree of trabeculation. Wu et al. were the first to note that sequences to evaluate late enhancement would help differentiate idiopathic dilated cardiomyopathy from ischemic dilated cardiomyopathy; they observed that all of the patients with ischemic dilated cardiomyopathy had ejection fractions of less than 30%, whereas only 12% of those with idiopathic dilated cardiomyopathy had ejection fractions of less than 30%. Our patient had no late gadolinium enhancement. The coronary angiography performed after the cardiac MRI showed the absence of significant lesions and thus confirmed the diagnosis of nonischemic dilated cardiomyopathy. The patient was treated with ACE inhibitors, low-dose beta blockers, and diuretics, and the symptoms that led to consultation improved significantly in a few days.

Cardiac MRI Findings

Distolic 4-chamber view SSFP-FIESTA image shows significant dilatation of the left ventricle in diastole (Fig. 3.3.1). The same sequence in systole shows good contractility of the right ventricle in comparison to the left ventricle, which has greatly depressed contractility (Fig. 3.3.2).

The GRE delayed enhancement sequence in four- and two-chamber views shows the absence of late gadolinium enhancement (Figs. 3.3.3 and 3.3.4).

Case 3.4

■

Interventricular Communication, Bicuspid Aortic Valve, and Aortic Coarctation

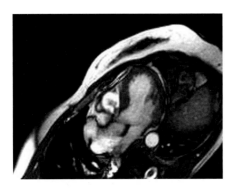

Fig. 3.4.1

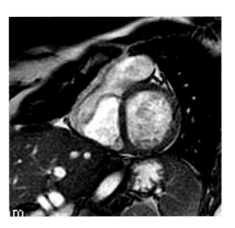

Fig. 3.4.2

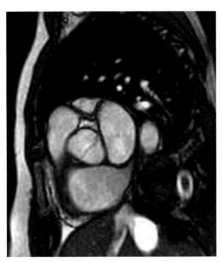

Fig. 3.4.3

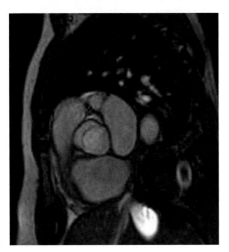

Fig. 3.4.4

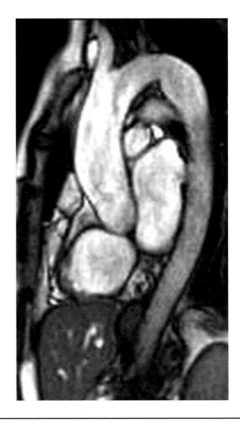

Fig. 3.4.5

A 32-year-old male patient with no relevant history was diagnosed with a heart murmur during childhood but had never undergone imaging tests until referred to a cardiologist after a routine physical examination at work. This patient had no shortness of breath or any other symptoms. Echocardiography showed a subaortic interventricular communication together with a bicuspid but normally functioning aortic valve. No other alterations were seen at echocardiography and the patient was referred for cardiac MRI to rule out the possibility of other associated congenital anomalies.

Introduction

Congenital heart defects are a group of structural heart malformations present at birth. They range from asymptomatic lesions that often remain undiagnosed until adulthood to very complex malformations that require surgical correction in the neonatal period. The anatomical and functional study of this type of condition can be very complex and may require a diagnostic imaging technique that can provide accurate, reproducible morphological and functional information. Thus, the first-line approach is echocardiography, and depending on the anomalies found and their complexity, cardiac MRI may be recommended. The main advantages of cardiac MRI in comparison to echocardiography are its wide field of view and excellent spatial resolution, which provide very detailed anatomical information in children as well as in adults. Moreover, cardiac MRI is considered the technique of choice for the evaluation of right ventricular function, which needs to be thoroughly assessed in this kind of patients. In addition to the findings diagnosed at echocardiography, cardiac MRI also allowed us to study the morphology of the aorta in this patient, which, given its prognostic implications in patients with bicuspid aortic valves, requires detailed study. In this case, there was no dilatation of the aortic root or of the ascending aorta, but there was a small coarctation that had gone undetected at echocardiography as no gradient was found.

Cardiac MRI Findings

4-chamber and short axis views SSFP-FIESTA images show the turbulence of the right ventricle secondary to the small, restrictive, subaortic interventricular communication. The size and function of the right ventricle are normal (Figs. 3.4.1 and 3.4.2). The orthogonal aortic value view SSEP-FIESTA cine sequence in systolic and diastole, depict the bicuspid, but normally functioning, aortic valve (Figs. 3.4.3 and 3.4.4). Aortic arch view cine sequence shows the normal diameter of the ascending aorta and slight coarctation and post-stenotic dilatation at the beginning of the descending aorta (Fig. 3.4.5).

Case 3.5
■
Noncompaction Cardiomyopathy

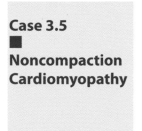

A 42-year-old female, previous smoker, without any personal or family history of interest was referred for study of recently diagnosed high blood pressure. The patient had no chest pain, dyspnea, palpitations, or syncope and was receiving medical treatment for hypertension.

The physical examination found no pulse asymmetry or abdominal murmur; heart auscultation showed rhythmic tones without splitting, murmurs, or rub. The remaining findings were within the normal limits. The EKG showed sinus rhythm with an isolated ventricular extrasystole, without criteria of left ventricular hypertrophy. At echocardiography, the right chambers, left atrium, and valves were normal; the left ventricle was not dilated, and no segmental alterations in contractility were observed. The apical and lateral views showed no left ventricular hypertrophy but raised suspicion for increased trabeculation; cardiac MRI was performed to evaluate possible noncompaction cardiomyopathy.

Introduction   Noncompaction or spongiform cardiomyopathy, recently renamed left ventricular noncompaction, was first described by Chin et al. in the early 1990s as the presence of trabeculae and recesses in the endocardium of the left ventricle.

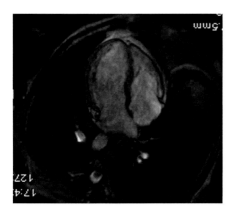

Fig. 3.5.1

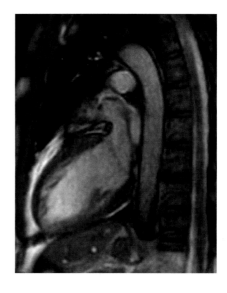

Fig. 3.5.2

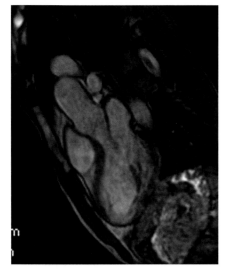

Fig. 3.5.3

The etiopathogeneis is due to an alteration in embryonic development. Initially, the myocardial wall is made up of a group of poorly organized muscular fibers with many trabeculae and recesses that provide nutrients to the tissues, similar to the myocardial walls of vertebrates other than mammals. During the sixth to eighth weeks of embryonic development, these structures become compacted from the epicardium to the endocardium, from the base to the apex, and from the septum to the lateral wall, coinciding with the beginning of coronary circulation.

The incidence of noncompaction cardiomyopathy is uncertain, and increased use of imaging techniques will help to clarify this issue. It is more common in males. Two presentations have been described: the isolated type and the familial type. Different genetic patterns have been described for the familial type and different genes involved have been identified (G4.5, FKB12, alpha-dystrobrevin).

The clinical presentation ranges from asymptomatic to major complications. The most common clinical presentations are heart failure, ventricular tachycardia, sudden death, cardioembolic events, and syncope. Other presentations commonly reported include ventricular extrasystoles, atrial fibrillation, and the more common presence of accessory pathways. Noncompaction cardiomyopathy has been frequently reported in association with neuromuscular diseases.

The best specific treatment is uncertain. Protocols similar to those used in cardiomyopathies (angiotensin-converting enzyme inhibitors, beta blockers, etc.) have been proposed. The use of salicylates to prevent cardioembolic events is widespread, although solid evidence for this practice is lacking. Prophylactic anticoagulation is not indicated, except in the presence of mural thrombosis or prior embolic events. Devices such as implanted cardioverter defibrillators are not indicated for prophylaxis except in sudden death survivors.

Previously, the prognosis was considered very poor, with a low 10-year survival rate, but the increased diagnosis of milder types is improving the prognosis. Due to the family association, family screening is clearly indicated for first-degree relatives.

Diagnostic criteria for noncompaction cardiomyopathy are:
- The presence of numerous trabeculae and prominent intratrabecular recesses, especially when located in the apex or in the medial segments of the ventricular myocardium.
- The visualization of blood flow in the recesses.
- A proportion of noncompacted to compacted myocardium >2 at echocardiography, and >2.3 at MRI (this cutoff yields sensitivity, specificity, and positive and negative predictive values of 86, 99, 75 and 99%, respectively).
- Some authors propose the absence of other heart defects, involvement of >50% of the entire chamber, or associated ventricular dysfunction, although there is no clear consensus regarding these criteria.

Cardiac MRI Findings

SSFP-FIESTA images show the left ventricle is not dilated or hypertrophic and its global and segmental contractility is conserved. Myocardial noncompaction is observed at the apical, anterior, lateral, posterior, and inferior levels, fulfilling the diagnostic criteria for noncompaction cardiomyopathy (ratio of noncompacted myocardium to compacted myocardium of 2.4 at the apical level) in the four-chamber view (Fig. 3.5.1), two-chamber view (Fig. 3.5.2), and the three-chamber view (Fig. 3.5.3).

Case 3.6
■
Supravalvular Pulmonary Stenosis

An overweighted 49-year-old woman with a history of dyslipemia due to hypercholesterolemia, menopause treated with estrogens, lower limb venous insufficiency, with no other relevant personal or family history, presented with shortness of breath on exertion (functional class I–II), without chest pain, dyspnea, palpitations, or syncope. In the physical examination, no pulse asymmetry or abdominal murmur was observed. Heart auscultation showed rhythmic tones, without splitting, grade II/VI harsh systolic murmur in the right parasternal region and in the base, without rub. The remaining findings were within normal limits. The EKG showed a sinus rhythm, without criteria of left or right ventricular hypertrophy. At echocardiography, the left atrium and left ventricle were normal, the right ventricle was not dilated, and contractility was conserved. The mitral valve was morphologically normal, without alterations in flow. The aortic valve was tricuspid and no alterations in flow were observed. The pulmonary valve was poorly seen, with apparently correct aperture. Although flow was turbulent with acceleration on Doppler imaging, stenosis was not clearly depicted. Cardiac MRI was performed to evaluate possible pulmonary (valvular or supravalvular) stenosis.

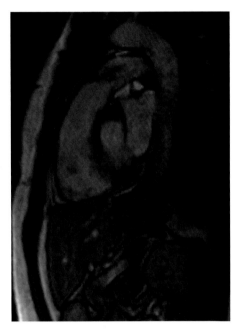

Fig. 3.6.1

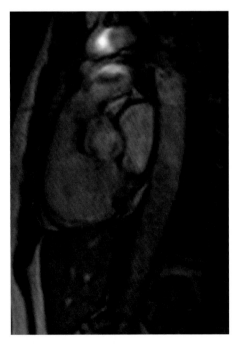

Fig. 3.6.2

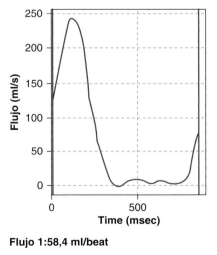

Flujo 1:58,4 ml/beat

Fig. 3.6.3

Pulmonary stenosis can occur in different locations: valvular, subvalvular, or supravalvular.

Valvular pulmonary stenosis can usually be evaluated correctly with transthoracic echocardiography. The evaluation of subvalvular or supravalvular obstruction can be more difficult, requiring transesophageal echocardiography or, more recently, cardiac MRI.

Subvalvular obstruction can affect the conus arteriosus (excessive hypertrophy or hypoplasia of the conus arteriosus) or may have a subinfundibular location (occasionally in adults with intraventricular communication due to hypertrophy of the septomarginal trabeculae, which cause medial ventricular obstruction, dividing the right ventricle into two chambers). Echocardiographic assessment of the parasternal region is difficult because the anomalous band can be mistaken for the normal moderator band, the jet from the obstruction can be confused with the jet from the intraventricular communication, the pressure gradient is underestimated (the jet is transversal to the ultrasonographic plane), and the increased systolic pressure of the right ventricle is attributed to pulmonary hypertension. Cardiac MRI enables the morphology of the subinfundibular obstruction to be determined with greater accuracy.

Adult patients with surgically treated congenital heart disease constitute another population that can be affected by subvalvular pulmonary stensosis. In these patients, stenosis of the right ventricular outflow tract can also be due to calcification of a prosthetic conduit, intrinsic degeneration of a biologic pulmonary prosthesis, or neointimal growth. Pulmonary prostheses can be properly assessed using echocardiography, but prosthetic conduits can be difficult to assess (conduits between the right ventricle and the pulmonary artery are often situated behind the sternum, in the high part of the chest). The use of MRI can obviate these difficulties and help to determine the site and cause of the obstruction.

Supravalvular pulmonary stenosis may occur in the pulmonary trunk or in the peripheral branches.

- Stenosis of the pulmonary trunk by a fibrous ring is uncommon but must be differentiated from valvular stenosis. Transthoracic echocardiography may suffice; however, doubts may arise regarding the precise location of the obstruction and its quantification. MR images are clearer.

In adults, the most frequent cause of stenosis of the pulmonary trunk is sequelae of pulmonary artery banding. Despite the resection of the band during the definitive repair of the heart defect, some patients continue to suffer from supravalvular pulmonary stenosis that can be assessed at echocardiography and/or MRI.

- Supravalvular stenosis located beyond the pulmonary bifurcation. This malformation can occur as an isolated anomaly; however, it more commonly occurs as a residue, sequela, or complication in patients operated on for tetralogy of Fallot or pulmonary atresia with an intraventricular shunt. Although suprasternal or transesophageal echocardiography can help to determine the morphology of the pulmonary branches, the imaging technique of choice is MRI. Three-dimensional reconstruction of gadolinium-enhanced MR angiography images of the pulmonary vessels provides a splendid image of the central pulmonary vascular tree.

Right outflow tract view SSFP-FIESTA images show turbulent flow approximately 12 mm above the plane of the pulmonary valve, with absence of dilatation of the pulmonary artery and the right ventricle (Figs. 3.6.1 and 3.6.2). The velocity-encoded cine MRI shows slightly elevated flow curve (Fig. 3.6.3), corresponding to mild supravalvular stenosis.

Introduction

Cardiac MRI Findings

Case 3.7

■

Agenesis of the Pericardium

An overweighted, dyslipemic 70-year-old woman with venous insufficiency due to bilateral saphenectomy and without other relevant history presented with occasional shortness of breath on considerable exertion and occasional palpitations. The physical examination showed symmetrical pulses, the absence of edemas, bilateral pulmonary ventilation, rhythmic cardiac auscultation, and a right parasternal diastolic murmur without rub or fremitus. EKG found SR with levorotation and horizontal axis, with no other relevant alterations. Chest X-ray showed slight leftward displacement of the cardiac silhouette without tracheal shift, lesions, or redistribution pattern. Echocardiography showed leftward heart displacement, no left ventricular dilatation or hypertrophy, preservation of global contractility, and paradoxical septal motion. The right chambers and the left atrium were not dilated. The mitral valve was morphologically normal, without dysfunction at Doppler imaging. The aortic valve had moderate regurgitation. The aortic root and ascending aorta were within normal limits.

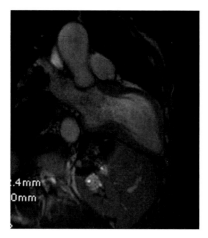

Fig. 3.7.1

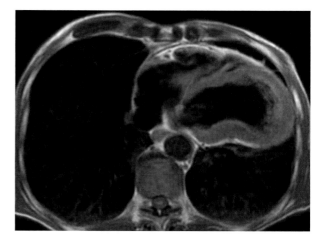

Fig. 3.7.2

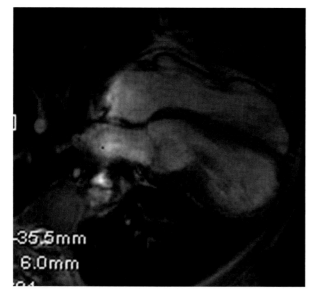

Fig. 3.7.3

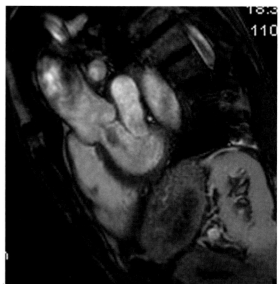

Fig. 3.7.4

Pericardial agenesis is a rare anomaly that was difficult to diagnose until the advent of high-quality MR images.

Pericardial agenesis originates from premature atrophy of the common cardinal vein, which impedes its normal closure. This explains the greater prevalence of the absence of the left hemipericardium (70%). Although total agenesis is the most common, partial agenesis also occurs. Pericardial agenesis is often associated with other alterations (bicuspid aortic valve, mitral stenosis, ductus, bronchogenic cyst, diaphragmatic hernia, and pectus excavatum).

Pericardial agenesis is generally asymptomatic, but fatigue, atypical precordial pain, heart failure, pericarditis, arrhythmias, peripheral embolism, syncope, and even sudden death have been reported. Partial agenesis can present myocardial herniation and strangulation with sudden death.

Although transthoracic or transesophageal echocardiography is not the technique of choice for the direct visualization of the pericardium, it can detect indirect, nonspecific signs such as anomalous position and motion of the heart, unusual acoustic window, paradoxical septal motion, hypermotility of the posterior wall, and anterior displacement of the left ventricle during systole.

CT enables the parietal pericardium to be visualized, but the left lateral and posterior portions are difficult to appreciate due to the different density of the mediastinal fat.

MRI is the technique of choice due to its greater discrimination among soft tissues and ability to acquire images in any plane. It enables the pericardium to be seen as a fine structure 1–2 mm thick situated between the epicardial fat and the mediastinal fat. MRI can also reveal situations involving risk, such as chamber herniation through partial defects or annular constriction of the ventricular myocardium, which is the most dangerous of these situations (the deaths reported in the literature presented partial agenesis in this area).

If direct visualization of the pericardium is not possible, it is useful to identify indirect diagnostic signs. In total left agenesis, these include laterodorsal heart displacement, contact between the left atrium and descending aorta, and the interpositioning of the lung parenchyma in the (absent) preaortic recess and the diaphragm, descending aorta, and diaphragmatic aspect of the heart. In partial absence of the left pericardium, indirect signs include the prominence of the left atrial appendage and normal location of the cardiac silhouette.

Complete or unilateral agenesis does not require treatment because these conditions do not involve any risks. Both symptomatic and asymptomatic partial agenesis that appears to involve the risk of ventricular strangulation on imaging techniques requires treatment.

SSFP-FIESTA (Figs. 3.7.1, 3.7.3, and 3.7.4) and black-blood (Fig. 3.7.2) images show partial pericardial agenesis at the anteroapical level that causes:

- Leftward displacement of the heart.
- Paradoxical septal motion; left ventricular contractility is normal.
- Normal right chambers.
- Moderate aortic regurgitation (Fig. 3.7.4) moderate degree regurgitating jet, with a ratio of the thickness of the jet related to the left ventricular outflow tract less than 50% and a regurgitation fraction of 40%. The mitral valve, the aortic root and ascending aorta are normal.

Case 3.8
■
Left Ventricular Hypertrophic Cardiomyopathy

A dyslipemic, overweighted, 47-year-old, male smoker with a family history of sudden death (grandfather at 66 years of age) presented with shortness of breath on exertion (moderate exertion, FC II), and occasional episodes of light-headedness without syncope. At physical examination, pulses were present and symmetrical. No edemas or jugular venous distension were found; auscultation was rhythmic with a systolic murmur in the base that increased with the Valsalva maneuver. EKG showed SR and criteria of ventricular hypertrophy and systolic overload. Echocardiography showed a nondilated left ventricle with severe concentric hypertrophy, acceleration of the outflow tract, no segmental alterations, and preservation of global contractility. The left atrium was dilated; the right chambers were normal. Mitral regurgitation due to systolic anterior motion (SAM) of the chords was present. The aortic valve opened correctly and had no transvalvular gradient.

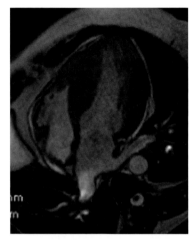

Fig. 3.8.1

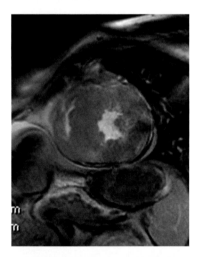

Fig. 3.8.2

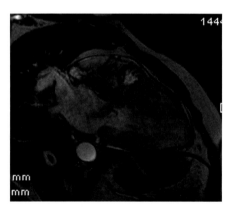

Fig. 3.8.3

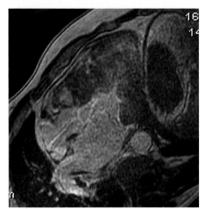

Fig. 3.8.4

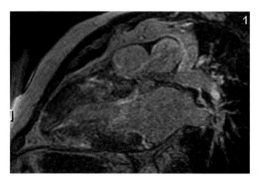

Fig. 3.8.5

Hypertrophic cardiomyopathy is characterized by inappropriate and unjustified myocardial hypertrophy (absence of systemic or cardiac causes that could justify it). The prevalence in adults is low (0.05–0.2%); the annual mortality rate in young people and children is 6%, hypertrophic cardiomyopathy is one of the most common causes of sudden death in adolescents. Approximately 50% of cases are hereditary (familial studies are indicated in newly diagnosed cases).

Histologically, it is characterized by hypertrophy of the myocytes with disarray and fibrosis.

Although the study of hypertrophic cardiomyopathy is based on echocardiography, which yields excellent results, magnetic resonance imaging (MRI) can provide additional information that can affect the prognosis.

Cardiac MRI makes it possible (a) to measure the mass and thickness of the myocardium, (b) to classify the pattern of myocardial distribution into asymmetrical septal, apical, or concentric, (c) to detect and quantify the presence of left ventricle outflow tract obstruction, (d) to detect the presence of anomalous anterior motion of the mitral valve or its chords, and (e) to detect and quantify the presence of mitral regurgitation. It also enables the extension and distribution of areas of fibrosis to be determined.

In hypertrophic cardiomyopathy, areas of late enhancement with gadolinium correspond to areas with scarring and disarray. Different patterns of both the extension and the distribution of late enhancement have prognostic implications. The patterns reported include diffuse involvement, predominantly trans-septal or septal right ventricle location, and focal patterns located in the ventricular junction, multifocal patterns, and, rarely, very near the subendocardial layer.

The extent of late myocardial enhancement correlates with the thickness of the ventricular wall, progressive ventricular dilatation, and ventricular systolic function; it is also associated to increased risk of sudden death (the relative risk can be doubled in cases with extensive and diffuse late myocardial enhancement).

The study of delayed gadolinium enhancement is also useful for checking the outcome of septal ablation or after myectomy, and for the differential diagnosis with some secondary cardiomyopathies that course with hypertrophy and characteristic gadolinium uptake (amyloidosis, Fabry disease, etc.).

Cardiac MRI Findings

4-chamber and short axis view SSFP-FIESTA images show severe concentric hypertrophy of the left ventricle (ventricular mass of 348 g), with a nondilated cavity and preserved global and segmental contractility (EF 73.8%) (Figs. 3.8.1 and 3.8.2). There is outflow tract acceleration with SAM of the chords of the mitral valve, leading to associated mitral regurgitation (Fig. 3.8.3).

4-chamber and long axis views GRE delayed enhancement images show a pattern of very extensive diffuse intramyocardial involvement (Figs. 3.8.4 and 3.8.5). The left atrium is moderately dilated (53 mm) and the right ventricle is hypertrophic, with an apical distribution. The mitral valve is thin with moderate mitral regurgitation due to SAM of the chords (Fig. 3.8.3).

Case 3.9
■
Left Ventricular Hypertrophy and Noncompaction Cardiomyopathy

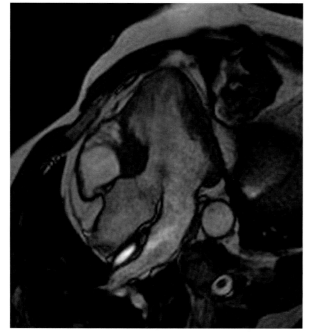

Fig. 3.9.1

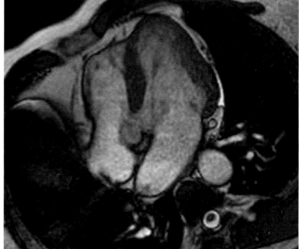

Fig. 3.9.2

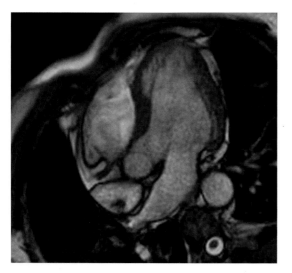

Fig. 3.9.3

A 52-year-old male smoker with peripheral vessel disease consulted for shortness of breath on exertion in FC II. The physical examination found pulses present and symmetrical, no edemas, no jugular venous distension, rhythmic auscultation, and no murmurs or rub. The ECG showed SR, with signs of ventricular hypertrophy and systolic overload. Echocardiography showed predominantly septal concentric hypertrophy of the left ventricle, no segmental alterations, and preserved global contractility. The left atrium was not dilated, and the right chambers were normal. Mitral valve function was normal; the aortic valve opened correctly and had no transvalvular gradient.

Introduction

Hypertrophic cardiomyopathy has been described in case 3.8 and noncompaction cardiomyopathy in case 3.5.

Only some isolated cases of left ventricular hypertrophy associated to noncompaction cardiomyopathy have been reported. It is unclear if there are mixed forms of both cardiomyopathies.

The prevalence, significance, and prognosis of this association are uncertain. Noncompaction can accompany hypertrophic or dilated myocardiopathies. The prognosis depends on the hypertrophic cardiomyopathy rather than the noncompaction of the left ventricle.

The diagnosis was oriented toward concentric hypertrophy and the cardiac MRI showed the association between concentric hypertrophic cardiomyopathy and noncompaction of the apical territories.

Cardiac MRI Findings

SSFP-FIESTA (Figs. 3.9.1–3.9.3) images show nondilated left ventricle with preserved global and segmental contractility, mild concentric hypertrophy (12 mm), more pronounced at the level of the basal septum, meeting criteria for severe hypertrophy (22 mm), and also at the level of the papillary muscles, with an insertion that reaches the base of the anterior aspect of the mitral ring.

At the same time, multiple trabeculae and recesses are seen in the apical and lateroapical myocardium, fulfilling the criteria for myocardial noncompaction. The left atrium and right chambers are not dilated.

Case 3.10
■
Arrhythmogenic Right Ventricular Dysplasia

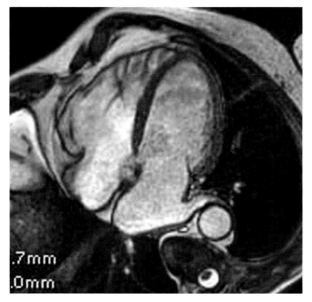

Fig. 3.10.1

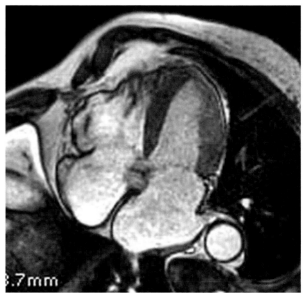

Fig. 3.10.2

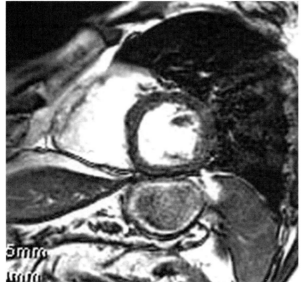

Fig. 3.10.3

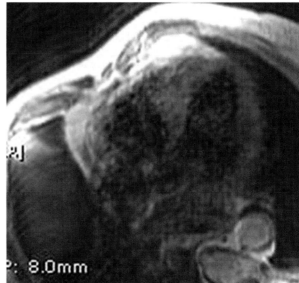

Fig. 3.10.4

A 40-year-old male patient with no relevant prior history presented with a 2-month history of palpitations followed by presyncope that resolved spontaneously. ECG showed an epsilon wave in the precordial derivations; Holter examination revealed multiple extrasystoles with episodes of self-limiting wide QRS tachycardia. Electrocardiography showed dilatation of the right chambers and a hypokinetic right ventricle. The patient underwent cardiac MRI for high suspicion of arrhythmogenic right ventricular dysplasia.

Introduction

Arrhythmogenic right ventricular dysplasia is a rare hereditary (autosomal dominant) cardiomyopathy that has aroused growing interest in recent years. It is difficult to diagnose, complex to treat, and potentially lethal. Arrhythmogenic right ventricular dysplasia is characterized by the specific involvement of the myocardium of the right ventricle, which atrophies and is replaced by fibrous or fibrofatty tissue, causing ventricular arrhythmias and progressive right heart failure. The ideal diagnostic method would be genetic analysis; however, genetic analysis is not available in routine daily practice and it only assesses the risk of developing this cardiomyopathy and not the degree of involvement. Endomyocardial biopsy has a low sensitivity (67%) due to the patchy distribution of the disease, so it is not routinely recommended. Cardiac MRI is considered the first choice noninvasive imaging technique to evaluate this disease because it can characterize the tissues as well as provide functional information about the right ventricle. The major diagnostic criteria are: (1) severe dilatation and decreased injection fraction of the right ventricle; (2) localized telediastolic aneurysms of the right ventricle; (3) severe segmental dilatation of the right ventricle; and (4) fatty deposits in the myocardium of the right ventricle. In advanced cases, there may be left ventricle involvement and the patient may present clinical signs and symptoms of biventricular cardiac insufficiency. Implanting automatic defibrillators to prevent sudden death has proven to be the most effective treatment.

Radiological Findings

End-diastolic and end-systolic 4-chamber view SSFP-FIESTA images show the dilatation of the right ventricle with telediastolic aneurysms in its base, as well as right ventricular dysfunction (Fig.3.10.1 and Fig. 3.10.2). The short-axis view SSFP-FIESTA sequence shows the dilatation of the right ventricle (Fig. 3.10.3). T1-weighted fast spin-echo four-chamber view demonstrates fatty infiltration (Fig. 3.10.4).

Case 3.11
■
Nonviable Myocardium After Acute Myocardial Infarction

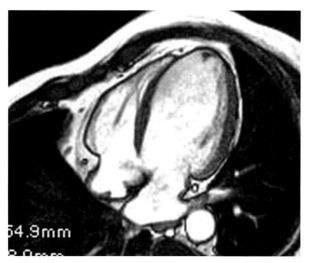

Fig. 3.11.1

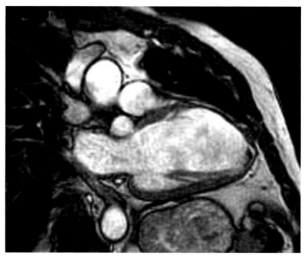

Fig. 3.11.2

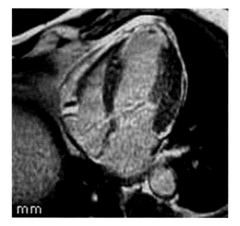

Fig. 3.11.3

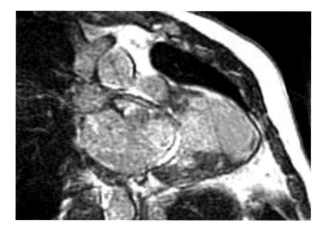

Fig. 3.11.4

A 79-year-old male patient with no known allergies to medications and the following cardiac risk factors: type II diabetes mellitus diagnosed 10 years prior and treated with oral antidiabetics, arterial hypertension treated with ACE inhibitors, smoking habit of 20 cigarettes per day, and peripheral vessel disease with intermittent claudication after 50 m. He was admitted to the emergency department 5 h after the onset of acute coronary syndrome with ST-elevation in the entire anterolateral aspect. The patient underwent fibrinolysis with tenecteplase. Once stabilized, the patient was transferred to a reference hospital and admitted to the coronary unit. Echocardiography showed extensive akinesia of the apical, medial septal, and anteromedial zones and an ejection fraction of 35%. Given the ventricular dysfunction, cardiac catheterization was performed; findings included a lesion in the medial portion of the anterior descending artery occluding 90% of the artery that was not susceptible to percutaneous revascularization; the distal vessel was suboptimal for surgical revascularization. Additional findings included lesions in the first and second marginal branches of the circumflex artery with 80% occlusion and very small distal vessels. No significant lesions were observed in the right coronary artery. Cardiac MRI was performed to assess viability as the patient was considered to have very high risk with the distal descending artery considered dubious for revascularization.

Introduction

Cardiac MRI has been established as the gold standard for the study of myocardial viability in routine clinical practice, both in the acute stage of the infarction and in chronic ischemic heart disease. Cardiac MRI provides various complementary perspectives in a single procedure that enable myocardial viability to be studied without the need for radiotracers. In the nonacute phase of infarction, late enhancement after gadolinium administration has proven to be the most accurate parameter for determining viability. Likewise, the absence of enhancement or a transmural extension of less than 50% in segments with severe contractile dysfunction have a sensitivity and specificity of 81 and 95%, respectively, in the diagnosis of viability. In regions with late enhancement above 75%, functional recovery after revascularization is very improbable. In segments with late enhancement between 50 and 75%, the response to low doses of dobutamine should be evaluated. Measuring the thickness of the nonenhancing myocardium (>3.9 mm) has also been shown to predict viability in a dysfunctional segment. In the present case, the myocardium was deemed unviable and the surgical option was considered futile.

Radiological Findings

4-chamber view SSFP-FIESTA image shows wall thinning at the level of the apex and of the medial septum, corresponding to akinetic zones (Fig. 3.11.1). The two-chamber view SSFP FIESTA sequence shows wall thinning at the level of the apex and of the anteromedial segment, corresponding to akinetic zones. The GRE delayed enhancement sequence images show the transmural signal in the nonviable apex and medial septum in the four-chamber view (Fig. 3.11.3) and in the apical and anteromedial segments in the two-chamber view (Fig. 3.11.4).

Case 3.12

■

Viable Myocardium After Acute Myocardial Infarction

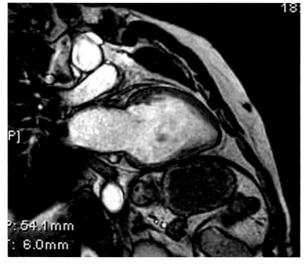

Fig. 3.12.1

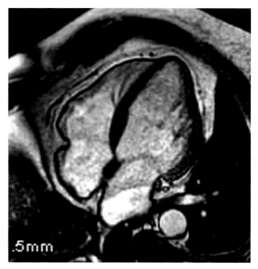

Fig. 3.12.2

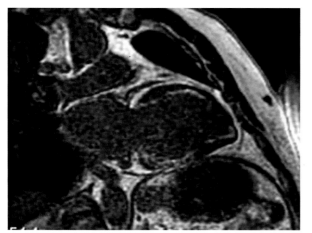

Fig. 3.12.3

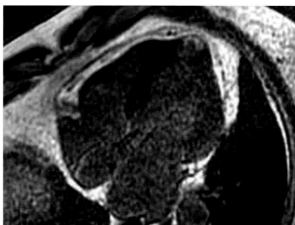

Fig. 3.12.4

A 72-year-old female patient with an allergy to penicillin, high blood pressure treated with calcium channel blockers, hypercholesterolemia treated with statins, long-standing type II diabetes mellitus with diabetic retinopathy treated with insulin, and chronic obstructive pulmonary disease with maximum expiratory volume per second of 40% treated with bronchodilators presented with acute coronary syndrome with persistent elevation of the ST segment in the inferior and posterior aspects of 2 h evolution. The patient was treated with fibrinolysis using tenecteplase; 48 h later the patient presented a new episode of typical angina pain without changes in the EKG that ceased a few minutes after the sublingual administration of nitroglycerine. Coronary angiography found severe disease in three vessels with calcification of the proximal third that was not susceptible to percutaneous revascularization. There was a 100% lesion in the proximal anterior descending artery but the distal vessel was doubtful for surgery and fed by collateral vessels from the right coronary artery. The circumflex artery had multiple 70–80% lesions in its proximal and medial portions; the distal vessel was in good condition. The echocardiogram showed an ejection fraction of 38% with inferobasal, posterobasal, and apical akinesia, as well as very severe anterior hypokinesia. Gadolinium-enhanced cardiac MRI was performed to assess the viability of the myocardium, especially of the territory fed by the anterior descending artery, because the patient was at especially high risk and had an anterior descending artery that was suboptimal for revascularization.

Introduction

In clinical practice, viable myocardium refers to nonnecrotic heart muscle with reduced contraction as a consequence of acute ischemia (stunned myocardium) or chronic ischemia (hibernating myocardium) that can be reversed with the normalization of myocardial perfusion. Hibernating myocardium is defined as contractile dysfunction caused by a chronic disruption of coronary flow that leads to prolonged and sustained ischemia. In the present case, the acute coronary syndrome is located in the inferoposterior region, but the patient has very severe disease in all three vessels. The presence of an occluded anterior descending artery with a vessel that is difficult to revascularize and is fed by collateral vessels, together with the very severe hypokinesia in the territory that it irrigates, makes it mandatory to study the viability of the myocardium to ensure that restoring perfusion by revascularization will be efficient in this high-risk situation. As we will see, the anterior territory showed necrosis, but necrosis affected less than 50% of the myocardial thickness at the level of the subendocardium, so this territory was potentially viable.

Cardiac MRI Findings

SSFP-FIESTA images show thinning at the level of the inferobasal segment, with associated akinesia. Notice that the thickness of the myocardium is conserved at the anterior level in the two-chamber view (Fig. 3.12.1). The four-chamber view shows thinning at the apical level; the rest of the segments are normal (Fig. 3.12.2). Two-chamber view GRE delayed enhancement sequence image shows late enhancement with gadolinium uptake greater than 75% at the inferobasal and apical levels (not viable) and less than 50% involving the basal interrior wall (Fig. 3.12.3). The four-chamber view GRE delayed enchancement sequence, shows an area of focal transmural enhancement at the level of the apex (Fig. 3.12.4).

Case 3.13
■
Double Aortic Lesion

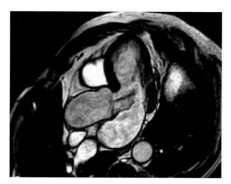

Fig. 3.13.1

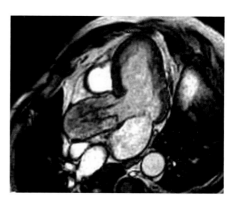

Fig. 3.13.2

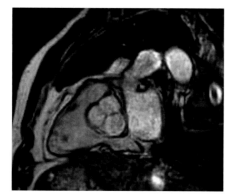

Fig. 3.13.3

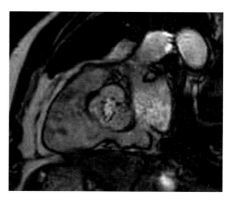

Fig. 3.13.4

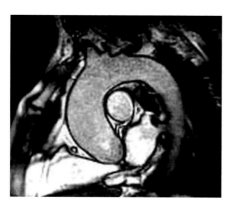

Fig. 3.13.5

A morbidly obese 70-year-old female patient with high blood pressure, dyslipemia, and chronic bronchitis consulted for shortness of breath on mild exertion of several months' evolution. The physical examination showed a systolic murmur with an aortic focus that was difficult to evaluate. The baseline EKG was normal. An echocardiogram was requested to rule out severe valve disease that might explain the dyspnea. However, as this was a very obese patient with possible chronic obstructive pulmonary disease, the very deficient acoustic window did not enable the valves to be correctly assessed and cardiac MRI was recommended.

Introduction

Echocardiography is the technique of choice for the detection and quantification of valvular defects. In cases in which a thorough echocardiographic study is impossible due to different factors that hinder correct visualization, cardiac MRI can provide complete and useful information, especially regarding pulmonary and aortic involvement (study of the large vessels, evaluation of the morphology of the aortic valve, quantification of ventricular hypertrophy and function). The main method for evaluating the severity of an aortic stenosis is to calculate the maximum velocity of blood flow using phase-contrast sequences and to calculate the gradient using Bernoulli's equation. Furthermore, cardiac MRI enables noninvasive visualization of the morphology and area of aperture. The best way to assess the degree of aortic insufficiency is to calculate the regurgitation fraction in phase-contrast sequences in planes perpendicular to the aortic valve. This is especially useful when the regurgitation is associated to aortic involvement, because the aortic diameters, the morphology of the valves, and the ventricular volumes can all be determined in the same examination, which helps in deciding the optimal time for surgery. In the present patient, both aortic lesions were mild, with a regurgitation fraction of 19% and an aortic area of 1.5 cm^2 with a maximum gradient of 30 mmHg; thus, the shortness of breath that led to the consultation was attributed solely to the patient's obesity and lung disease.

Cardiac MRI Findings

SSFP-FIESTA images show the low-grade aortic regurgitation jet in the three-chamber view of a long-axis slice (Fig. 3.13.1). The three-chamber view of a long-axis plane shows the degree of aperture of the aortic valve (Fig. 3.13.2). Orthogonal aortic valve SSFP-FIESTA cine sequence in diastole shows that the valve is tricuspid and in telesystole shows that the degree of stenosis is mild (Figs. 3.13.3 and 3.13.4). Aortic arch view cine sequence shows moderate dilatation of the ascending aorta, measuring 44 mm of maximum diameter (Fig. 3.13.5).

Case 3.14

■

Aneurysmal Dilatation of the Pulmonary Artery

An 80-year-old woman with a history of high blood pressure, dyslipemia, mild renal insufficiency (renal clearance 45 cc/min), and degenerative arthropathy limiting her ability to walk, complained of shortness of breath on exertion. Mediastinal widening was noted during the preoperative work-up for hip replacement surgery. Physical examination showed that pulses were present and symmetrical, and found subedemas, slight jugular ingurgitation, and grade 2/6 right parasternal systolic murmurs. EKG showed SR and incomplete right bundle branch block. Echocardiography found no dilatation or hypertrophy of the left ventricle and preservation of global and segmental contractility. The left atrium was not dilated; the right ventricle was dilated, with preserved contractility. The mitral valve was morphologically normal and without dysfunction at Doppler imaging. No tricuspid insufficiency was observed. The ascending aorta was dilated.

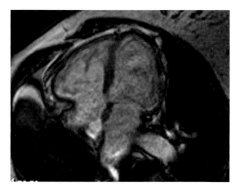

Fig. 3.14.1

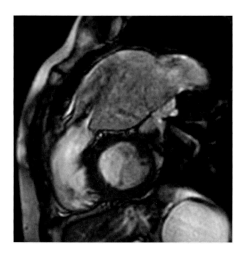

Fig. 3.14.2

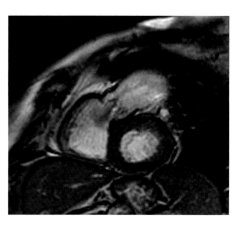

Fig. 3.14.3

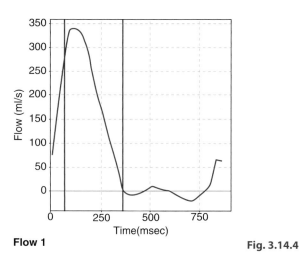

Flow 1

Fig. 3.14.4

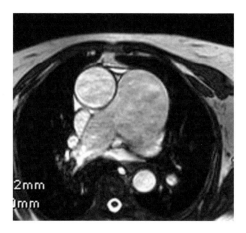

Fig. 3.14.5

Aneurysm of the pulmonary artery, defined as dilatation of the pulmonary artery or its branches to greater than 4 cm, is very uncommon.

The causes are not well understood. Half of all cases are associated to congenital heart disease (most commonly patent ductus arteriosus, followed by interatrial and interventricular communication), all of which are usually associated to pulmonary hypertension. Other, noncongenital, causes include infections (syphilis, endocarditis, tuberculosis, etc.), arteriosclerosis, degenerative changes in the medial layer, vasculitis, and trauma. A number of unexplained cases have been classified as idiopathic.

A wide variety of cases have been reported, including single and multiple, saccular or fusiform, central (truncal) or peripheral aneurysms. Findings at histology include cystic medial necrosis, arteriosclerotic changes, and loss of elastic fibers.

Generally, pulmonary artery aneurysms have no clinical manifestations and are incidental findings at imaging. Nonspecific symptoms, like dyspnea, chest pain, right heart failure, and hemoptysis (which suggest instability and indicate surgery) have been reported.

MRI and CT are the diagnostic techniques of choice, and angiography is reserved for surgical cases or therapeutic procedures. Echocardiography enables the diagnosis and study of associated structural anomalies of the heart.

The prognosis is unclear. Idiopathic aneurysms and those associated to low pulmonary pressure are considered benign and have a low rate of dissection or rupture. Rather than the diameter of the aneurysm, the follow-up and treatment depend on other parameters, such as the degree of pulmonary hypertension, the diameter and contractility of the right ventricle (as a consequence of pulmonary regurgitation), associated congenital pathology, or the etiology.

The treatment of pulmonary artery aneurysm can be medical or surgical. Medical treatment is indicated in cases with benign prognosis; it consists of periodic examination and controlling pulmonary hypertension. Recent reports describe some cases of aneurysms associated to Behçet's disease that responded to treatment with immunosuppressors. Surgical treatment is indicated for unstable aneurysms, cases with hemoptysis, and those considered at high risk of rupture and greater mortality (micotic aneurysms; those associated to Behçet's disease, Marfan syndrome, primary antiphospholipid syndrome, and a few others). The surgical technique depends on the location, number, and etiology of the aneurysms, and embolization is the treatment of choice in cases with more peripheral sites of vascular delatation.

Introduction

4-chamber view SSFP-FIESTA image (Figs. 3.14.1–3.14.3) shows the left ventricle is not dilated or hypertrophic, and global and segmental contractility are preserved. The right ventricle is slightly dilated but maintains good global contractility. (Fig. 3.14.1). In the right outflow tract view SSFP-FIESTA sequence, the tricuspid pulmonary valve with dome-shaped aperture shows a double lesion, with moderate stenosis (Figs. 3.14.2) and moderate regurgitation (Fig. 3.14.3) as demonstrated in the flow/time curve obtained from the pulmonary valve velocity-encoded phase-contrast MRI sequence (Fig. 3.14.4). There is a large, aneurysmal dilatation of the pulmonary artery (maximum diameter 68 mm) (Fig. 3.14.5).

Cardiac MRI Findings

Case 3.15
■
Acute Myocarditis

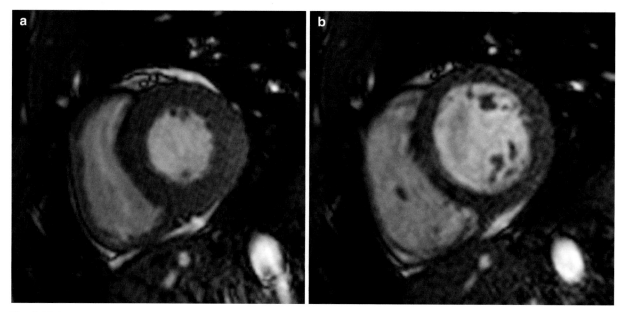

Fig. 3.15.1

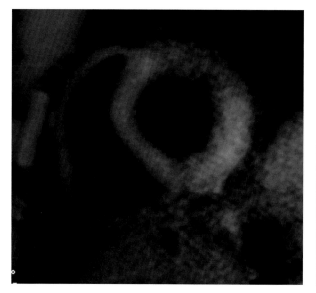

Fig. 3.15.2

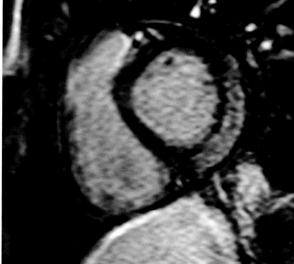

Fig. 3.15.3

A 16-year-old male without cardiovascular risk factors presented to the emergency room with precordial pain of sudden onset, clinically indistinguishable from acute myocardial infarction. ST segment elevation in the inferolateral wall was observed. Peak serum creatine kinase and T-troponin levels were elevated.

Comments

Myocarditis is a group of diseases with infectious, toxic, and autoimmune etiologies that is characterized by inflammation of the heart and myocyte necrosis. Subsequent myocardial destruction can lead to dilated cardiomyopathy. The true incidence of myocarditis is unknown because many cases are asymptomatic and there is no clear diagnostic algorithm. Acute myocarditis can be confused with acute infarction, and rarely, it can be fulminant. An antecedent viral syndrome is present in more than half of patients with myocarditis. Endomyocardial biopsy is still considered the "gold standard," although its reported sensitivity is limited due to the focal nature of the disease. Diagnosis in the acute phase relies more commonly on electrocardiographic alterations and elevation of cardiac enzymes.

MRI is the imaging technique of choice for the evaluation of myocarditis. Like echocardiography, MRI enables evaluation of global and regional left ventricular function. MRI is the only imaging technique that can identify myocardial edema or delayed enhancement, which typically show a subepicardial distribution. Delayed enhancement related to myocardial ischemia is most commonly subendocardial. MRI can be used to guide endomyocardial biopsy, increasing its accuracy.

MRI Findings

Figure 3.15.1 (a, b) Balanced fast field-echo cine MRI images obtained in the short-axis at end-systole and end-diastole, respectively, show mild hypokinesia of the inferolateral wall. Left ventricle ejection fraction was 65%.

Figure 3.15.2 Short-axis STIR black-blood-sequence shows subepicardial edema in the inferolateral wall.

Figure 3.15.3 Three-dimensional double inversion T1-weighted fast field-echo late enhancement sequence obtained in the short axis shows subepicardial enhancement in the same distribution as in the segmental wall motion abnormality and the myocardial edema.

Case 3.16

Aortic Coarctation

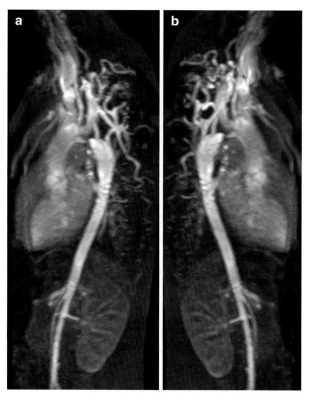

Fig. 3.16.1

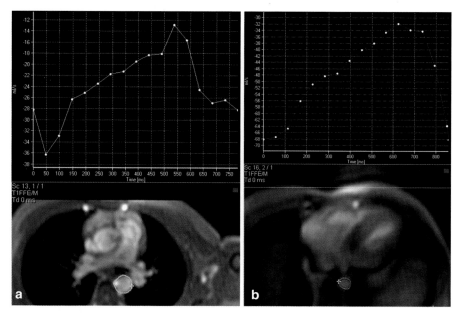

Fig. 3.16.2

A 10-year-old male presented high blood pressure and dyspnea; MRI was indicated to rule out aortic coarctation.

Coarctation of the aorta consists of an infolding of the posterolateral wall of the aorta at the level of the ligamentum arteriosum, with secondary narrowing of the aortic lumen. There are two main types, according to its location:
- Preductal coarctation, which occurs proximal to the ligamentum arteriosum and is normally discovered in infants.
- Postductal coarctation, the most common type, which occurs distal to the ligamentum and the origin of the left subclavian artery and rarely shows symptoms in childhood.

Conditions associated to aortic coarctation are: hypoplasia of the aortic arch, bicuspid aortic valve, patent ductus arteriosus, ventricular septal defect, tricuspid atresia, mitral valve abnormalities, berry aneurysms in the circle of Willis, and Turner's syndrome.

MRI is the imaging technique of choice for the evaluation of aortic coarctation. MR angiography can show the location, length, and severity of the stenosis as well as the development of collateral circulation. Velocity-encoded phase-contrast sequences allow the pressure gradient across the stenosis and blood volume through the collateral circulation to be quantified. Both measurements are crucial for clinical management, helping to decide whether to use observation and medical treatment or surgical treatment, or occasionally, balloon dilatation.

Figure 3.16.1 (a, b) Sagittal-oblique MIP reconstructions of a postcontrast aortic 3D MR angiogram show severe postductal aortic coarctation with extensive collateral circulation.

Figure 3.16.2 (a, b) Velocity-encoded phase contrast sequences immediately distal to the coarctation (a) and in the distal descending aorta (b) together with the corresponding flux (ml/s) /time (ms) curves. Blood volume at the distal thoracic aorta is increased (40 ml) compared to the postductal level (19 ml), indicating marked returning circulation through collateral circulation.

Case 3.17
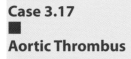
Aortic Thrombus

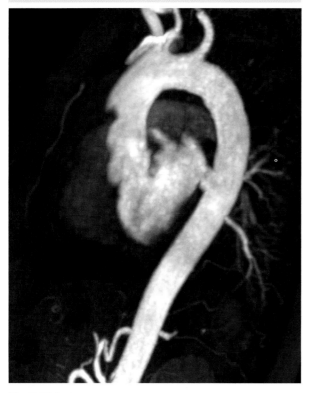

Fig. 3.17.1

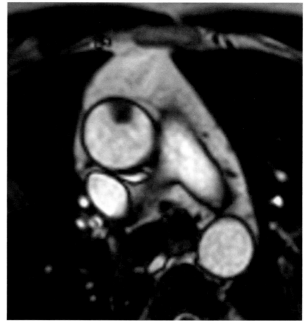

Fig. 3.17.2

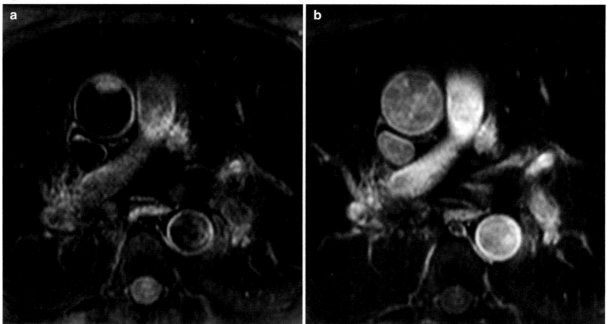

Fig. 3.17.3

A 50-year-old male without cardiovascular risk factors underwent transesophageal echocardiography in the work-up of atypical chest pain; a hypermobile mass was found in the ascending aorta, 5 cm above the aortic valve. MRI was performed for further characterization.

Comments

Aortic thrombi cause approximately 5% of peripheral arterial embolisms. The presence of thrombi in an atherosclerotic and/or aneurysmatic aorta with peripheral arterial embolism is common. However, thrombus formation in a morphologically normal aorta is rare, especially in the absence of trauma, infection, or other prothrombotic risk factors, such as hypercoagulability, antiphospholipid syndrome, disorders of proteins C or S, or vasculitis. Aortic thrombi most commonly occur in the distal abdominal aorta.

New imaging techniques, such as multislice CT, MRI, and transesophageal echocardiography, have enabled aortic thrombi to be detected with increasing frequency. MRI can reliably rule out aortic wall involvement and make it possible to reach a specific diagnosis. The absence of enhancement rules out neoplastic lesions. The signal characteristics of thrombi depend on their age: acute thrombi are hyperintense on T1- and T2-weighted sequences, subacute thrombi show decreased signal intensity on T2-weighted images, and chronic thrombi are markedly hypointense on all sequences.

Diverse treatments, including anticoagulant therapy, thrombolysis, thromboaspiration, and surgery have been used with variable success. Endovascular stent-grafting is a new minimally invasive therapy.

MRI Findings

Figure 3.17.1 Sagittal MIP reconstruction of a postcontrast 3D high resolution gradient-echo MR angiogram shows a nodular endoluminal defect in the anterior wall of the ascending aorta.

Figure 3.17.2 Axial balanced fast field-echo sequence shows a hypointense endoluminal nodule in the anterior wall of the ascending aorta.

Figure 3.17.3 (a, b) Pre- and post-contrast axial black-blood fat-suppressed T1-weighted sequences demonstrate mild hyperintensity of the thrombus and absence of enhancement.

Case 3.18
■
Chiari Network

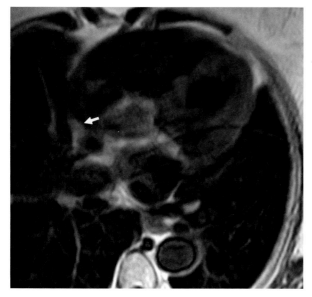

Fig. 3.18.1

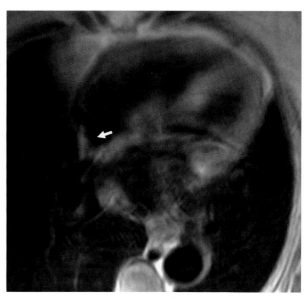

Fig. 3.18.2

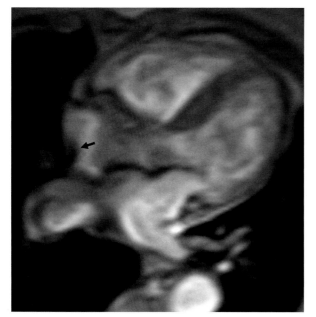

Fig. 3.18.3

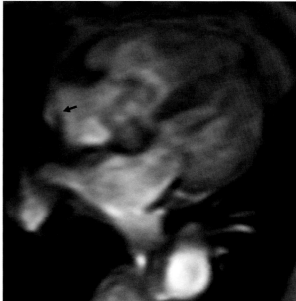

Fig. 3.18.4

A 73-year-old woman underwent MRI to characterize an endocavitary mass in the posterior wall of the right atrium discovered incidentally at transthoracic echocardiography.

The fibromuscular elements of the posterior wall of the right atrium, including the crista terminalis, Chiari network, and eustachian valve, are embryologic remnants of incomplete regression. These elements are common pitfalls for right atrium masses in echocardiography and in the MRI diagnosis of intracavitary tumors. They appear as a nodule of variable size isointense to myocardium in all pulse sequences. Their typical location can help ensure that they are recognized so they should never be mistaken for a cardiac tumor or thrombus. MRI is the imaging technique of choice for the evaluation of intracavitary tumors.

Figures 3.18.1 and 3.18.2 Consecutive axial black-blood proton density-weighted images show a nodular thickening of the posterior wall of the right atrium, which looks likes an endocavitary mass.

Figures 3.18.3 and 3.18.4 Consecutive four-chamber view balanced fast field-echo images confirm the endocavitary nodular thickening connected to a linear structure, which was mobile on cine sequences. These are typical features of the Chiari network.

Case 3.19

◼ Ischemic Dilated Cardiomyopathy

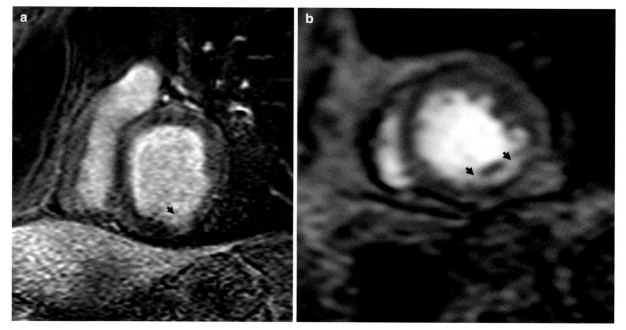

Fig. 3.19.2

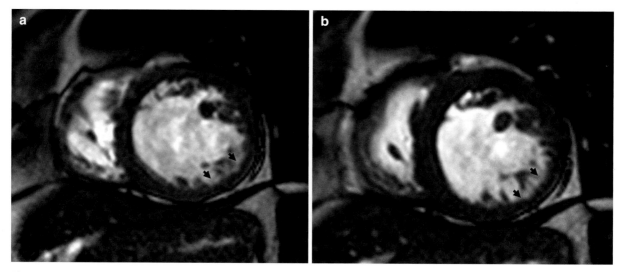

Fig. 3.19.1

An obese 57-year-old male smoker showed progressive clinical signs of heart failure. There were no EKG signs or clinical history of ischemic heart disease. Echocardiography showed systolic dysfunction and dilatation of the left ventricle.

Dilated cardiomyopathy (DCM) is characterized by progressive dilatation of the heart with loss of contractile function. Histologically, it is characterized by interstitial fibrosis with a decrease in contractile myocytes and, in the late stages, wall thinning. Although echocardiography is the standard tool in the evaluation of left ventricle size and function in patients with DCM, MRI is more reproducible; moreover, it allows changes in wall thickness to be analyzed, impaired fiber shortening to be measured, and end-systolic wall stress to be calculated. End-systolic wall stress is a very sensitive parameter for detecting changes in left ventricular function. MRI can also assess right ventricle and atrial volumes and function, which may be involved in DCM. As MRI has proven very sensitive in the detection of subtle changes in left ventricle function, it is appropriate for monitoring the response to treatment for DCM.

MRI is able to distinguish between ischemic and nonischemic dilated cardiomyopathy. In the nonischemic types, left ventricular wall thickness is uniform, without areas of wall thinning. When DCM is caused by myocardial ischemia, there are areas of wall thinning, a decrease in number and size of the trabeculae, and sometimes ventricular aneurysms. Specific causes of dilated cardiomyopathy, such as hemochromatosis and myocarditis, can be identified with CMR. Delayed enhancement studies can show regional hyperenhancement in a variable number of causes of DCM. Although delayed enhancement patterns are nonspecific, subendocardial enhancement suggests an ischemic origin and subepicardial enhancement has recently been related to inflammatory causes, such as myocarditis.

Figure 3.19.1 (a, b) Short-axis cine balanced fast field-echo sequences obtained at end diastole and end-systole, respectively, show dilatation of the left ventricle with global systolic dysfunction. Note the myocardial thinning and akinesia of the inferolateral wall (*arrows*). Left ventricular ejection fraction was 33%.

Figure 3.19.2 (a, b) Short-axis late enhancement three-dimensional double inversion T1-weighted fast field-echo images at mid-ventricular and apical levels, respectively, reveal subendocardial late enhancement in the inferolateral wall that is highly suspicious for nonviable myocardium secondary to infarction. Mid-left circumflex coronary artery stenosis was confirmed at coronary angiography.

Case 3.20
■
Hematogenous Cardiac Metastasis

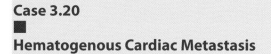

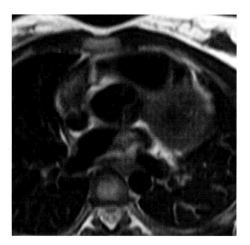

Fig. 3.20.1

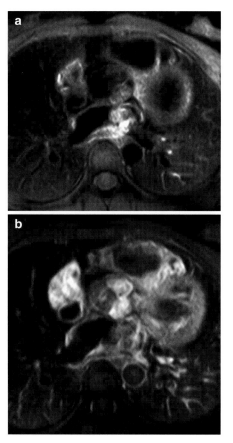

Fig. 3.20.3

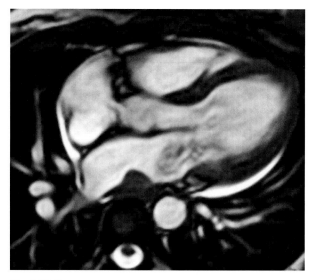

Fig. 3.20.2

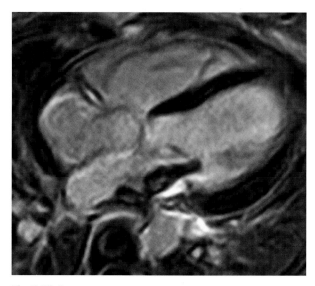

Fig. 3.20.4

A 56-year-old woman with a history of thyroid leiomyosarcoma in clinical remission underwent MRI to study an endocavitary mass in the left atrium discovered incidentally on follow-up CT.

Comments

Metastases to the heart and pericardium are much more common – from 20 to 100 times more prevalent – than primary cardiac tumors and are generally associated with a poor prognosis. Although secondary heart involvement is identified in one-fifth of all patients with metastatic cancer at autopsy, its clinical diagnosis has been much less common. The advent of multislice CT and, particularly, cardiac MRI have increased the radiological diagnosis of metastatic heart disease, and these imaging modalities, along with echocardiography, may be helpful in the management of oncologic patients with or without cardiac symptoms. MRI can also help in surgical planning and follow-up as well as in evaluating the response to radiotherapy or chemotherapy. Finally, MRI is also useful in the characterization of a cardiac mass or pericardial effusion in patients with a known extracardiac primary malignancy.

Neoplasms most likely to invade the heart and pericardium are melanoma, lymphoma, and cancers of the lung, breast, and esophagus. Metastatic disease can involve the heart by one of the four basic pathways: direct extension, lymphatic spread, hematogenous spread, and transvenous extension. Additionally, combined pathways, such as hematogenous lung metastases directly invading the heart and pericardium, are also possible.

MRI Findings

Figure 3.20.1 Axial black-blood T2-weighted TSE image shows a heterogeneous endocavitary mass with invasion of the lateral wall of the left atrium.

Figure 3.20.2 Four-chamber balanced phase field-echo sequence shows a parietal component of the posterior mass and another endocavitary component which protrudes through the mitral valve.

Figure 3.20.3 (a, b) Pre- and post-contrast axial black-blood fat-suppressed T1-weighted TSE images show a hyperintense mass with slight heterogeneous enhancement.

Figure 3.20.4 3D four-chamber delayed-enhancement double inversion phase-field echo sequence confirms the patchy enhancement of the tumor.

Case 3.21

■

Pericardial Cyst

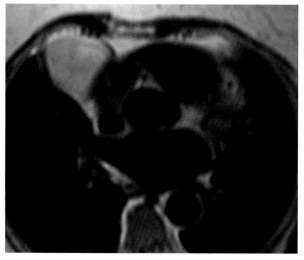

Fig. 3.21.1

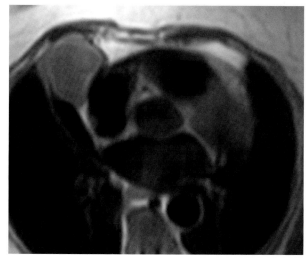

Fig. 3.21.2

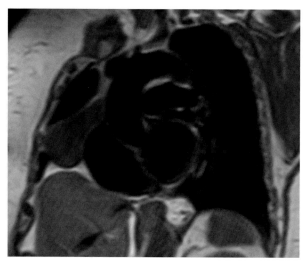

Fig. 3.21.3

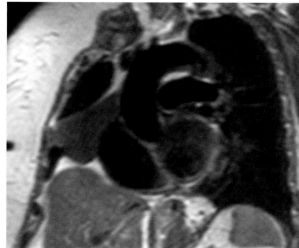

Fig. 3.21.4

A 67-year-old woman with an incidental right paracardiac mass on chest CT underwent MRI to characterize the mass.

Comments

Pericardial cysts are rare benign developmental abnormalities that are clinically indistinguishable from pericardial diverticula. They are most commonly located in the right cardiophrenic angle, although they can occur in any location adjacent to the pericardium. They are usually an incidental finding because they are asymptomatic masses. In rare cases pericardial cysts can cause a mass effect, leading to, for example, obstruction of the right ventricular outflow tract. When pericardial cysts are not located in the right cardiophrenic angle, they become indistinguishable from bronchogenic or thymic cysts.

Pericardial cysts are unilocular thin-walled structures strongly bound to the pericardium through either a pedicle or a broad implantation base. They usually contain transudates. In pericardial cysts that contain calcifications, CT can add valuable information over MRI. On MRI, they appear as cystic lesions: thin walled, homogeneous masses that are hypointense on T1-weighted images and hyperintense on T2-weighted images, without evident enhancement on postcontrast series. Occasionally, pericardial cysts present a highly proteinaceous content and, therefore, their signal intensity on T1-weighted images increases. In children, pericardial cysts may be mistaken for pericardial teratomas.

MRI Findings

Figures 3.21.1 and 3.21.2 Axial black-blood T2-weighted and T1-weighted TSE images, respectively, show a right paracardiac mass connected to the pericardium at the level of the right appendage that is hyperintense on both sequences. High signal intensity on the T1-weighted image reveals its mucinous content.

Figures 3.21.3 and 3.21.4 Pre- and post-contrast coronal black-blood T1-weighted TSE images, respectively, demonstrate the absence of enhancement of the mass and its broad-based connection to the pericardium.

Case 3.22

■

True Ventricular Apical Aneurysm of Ischemic Origin Associated to Acute Thrombus

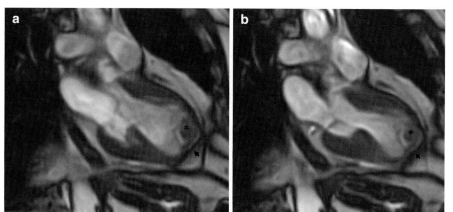

Fig. 3.22.1

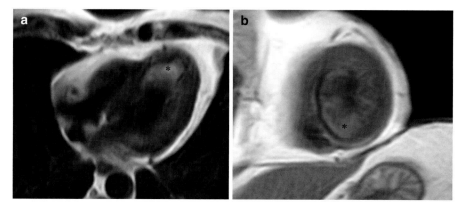

Fig. 3.22.2

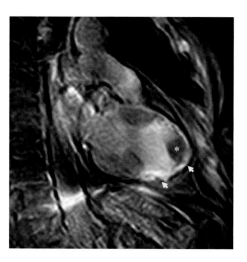

Fig. 3.22.3

An obese 64-year-old male smoker with a previous apical myocardial infarct showed increasing focal dilatation and akinesia of the apex in consecutive echocardiograms.

Ventricular aneurysms are classified as congenital or acquired. Congenital left ventricular aneurysms are rare and typically present in young black adults. They may produce an abnormal bulging in the left atrium or present as cardiac enlargement secondary to aortic insufficiency.

Acquired aneurysms may be true or false aneurysms. Both types usually occur secondary to myocardial infarction. Clinically, they are usually associated to persistent congestive heart failure, arrhythmias, and peripheral embolization. True ventricular aneurysms are localized outpouchings of the ventricular wall, associated to dyskinesia, that have a wide-mouthed connection with the left ventricle. They produce paradoxical expansion during systole. They are most commonly located in the anterolateral or apical wall and commonly present in association with a thrombus. They rarely rupture and may have fibrotic or calcified walls.

False aneurysms or pseudoaneurysms occur after left ventricle rupture into the pericardial sac contained by pericardial adhesions. They are a rare complication of myocardial infarction and occasionally have a posttraumatic origin. They lack a true myocardial wall, and their connection with the ventricular lumen is usually smaller than in true aneurysms. False aneurysms are most frequently located in the posterolateral wall and have a high risk of rupture.

Left ventricular angiography and echocardiography are the most widely used imaging techniques in the evaluation of left ventricular aneurysms. Angiography is invasive with associated risks, such as pseudoaneurysm rupture or displacement of a thrombus. Echocardiography is often limited in the evaluation of the left ventricular apex, where the majority of aneurysms are located. Therefore, MRI is the technique of choice for the evaluation of ventricular aneurysms, as its multiplanar capabilities make it possible to locate the lesion, to determine whether a myocardial wall is present, and to obtain complementary information such as the characteristic marked delayed enhancement of the pericardium in false aneurysms.

Figure 3.22.1 (a, b) Long-axis cine balanced fast field-echo images obtained at end-diastole and end-systole, respectively, show focal dilatation of the left ventricular apex with global systolic dysfunction. Note the myocardial thinning and akinesia of the apical wall (*arrows*). Left ventricular ejection fraction was 33%. An endocavitary hypointense mass attached to myocardial wall (*asterisks*) was identified, representing a thrombus.

Figure 3.22.2 (a) Four-chamber view black-blood T2-weighted TSE image and (b) short-axis view black-blood T1-weighted TSE image demonstrate hyperintensity on both sequences of the thrombus (*asterisks*), indicating its acute nature.

Figure 3.22.3 Late enhancement three dimensional double inversion fast field-echo T1-weighted image obtained in the long-axis reveals transmural enhancement of the wall of the apex (*arrows*), indicating nonviable myocardium secondary to previous infarct. Note the absence of enhancement of the thrombus (*asterisk*).

Case 3.23

■

Cardiac Amyloidosis

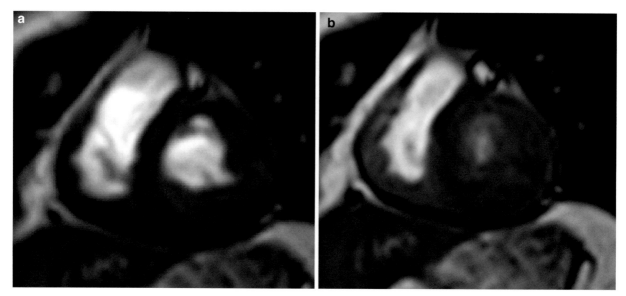

Fig. 3.23.1

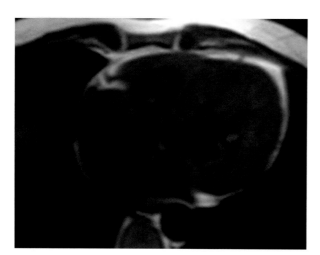

Fig. 3.23.2

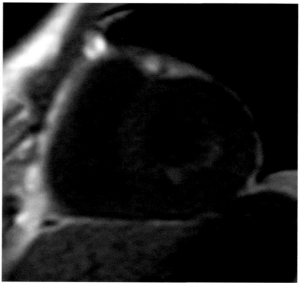

Fig. 3.23.3

A 63-year-old man with progressive clinical signs of left heart failure and infiltrative heart disease suspected at echocardiography underwent MRI for further evaluation.

Amyloidosis represents the deposition of nonsoluble proteinaceous material in different organs. Cardiac involvement can occur in most of the different subtypes of amyloidosis. Cardiac amyloid deposition is diffuse, and this makes it easy to diagnose by endomyocardial biopsy. Morphologically, cardiac amyloidosis produces diffuse cardiac thickening similar to that seen in hypertrophic cardiomyopathy, although functionally it presents with a restrictive pattern. The long-term prognosis is very poor after the onset of heart failure.

MRI is very useful in the evaluation of cardiac amyloidosis. First, MRI is the imaging technique of choice for the evaluation of the diastolic dysfunction typical of restrictive cardiomyopathies. A specific diagnosis of amyloidosis can be suspected based on the following features: biatrial dilatation with normal-sized ventricles, global ventricular contractile impairment, increased ventricular wall thickness, a significant decrease in myocardial signal on T1-weighted and T2-weighted black-blood sequences, and diffuse subendocardial late enhancement without a distribution typical for any particular vascular territory. Other associated findings are: systolic dysfunction, in advanced phases, and pericardial and pleural effusions.

Figure 3.23.1 (a, b) Balanced fast field-echo cine images obtained in the short-axis at end-diastole and end-systole, respectively, show diffuse thickening of the myocardium of both ventricles, although especially of the lateral and inferior walls of the left ventricle, as well as mild hypokinesia of the inferolateral wall. Note the diastolic dysfunction with absence of diastolic relaxation in the areas where the myocardial thickening is greatest. Left ventricular ejection fraction was 65%.

Figure 3.23.2 Four-chamber view black-blood T1-weighted image shows left ventricle thickening and decreased signal intensity of myocardium.

Figure 3.23.3 2D double inversion T1-weighted fast field-echo late enhancement sequence obtained in the short axis shows subendocardial enhancement in the same distribution as the myocardial thickening (inferolateral wall of the left ventricle).

Case 3.24
Fontan Conduit Evaluation

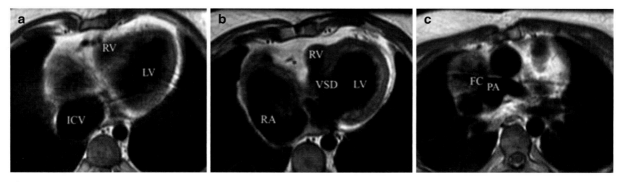

Fig. 3.24.1

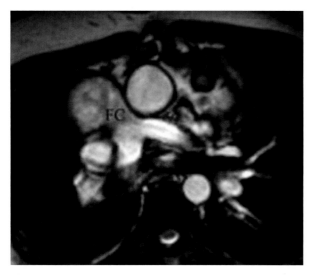

Fig. 3.24.2

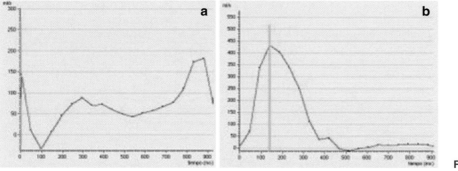

Fig. 3.24.3

A 24-year-old man with a history of tricuspid atresia corrected at age 6 presented with dyspnea on mild exertion. MRI was performed for follow up.

Comments

Fontan first described a surgical procedure for the treatment of tricuspid atresia in 1971. Different types of connections have been developed for the treatment of a heterogeneous group of congenital cardiac malformations characterized by a single systemic ventricle. A tunnel is created to direct systemic venous circulation into the pulmonary arterial circuit. The types of connection are classified as cavopulmonary, atriopulmonary, and atrioventricular connection.

Before surgery, it is important to assess the function and morphology of the systemic ventricle, as left ventricular systolic function can worsen in the first 2 years after the Fontan procedure. Another common postsurgical complication is obstruction of the conduit. Minimal adequate Fontan conduit diameter in the axial plane is considered 20 mm. Phase contrast sequences allow direct calculation of the pressure gradient in the conduit to rule out obstruction. The McGoon ratio is a useful indicator of Fontan conduit dysfunction. This ratio is obtained by summing the diameter of the distal right and left pulmonary arteries and dividing by the diameter of the descending aorta; values below 1.8 indicate Fontan conduit dysfunction.

MRI is the imaging technique of choice for the evaluation of surgically treated congenital cardiomyopathies. In patients with a Fontan conduit, black-blood sequences enable morphological assessment of the systemic ventricle, associated malformations, and diameter of the conduit. Permeability of the Fontan conduit must be evaluated with enhanced angiography and phase contrast imaging, which also allows the flow pattern to be identified and the pressure gradient through the conduit to be calculated.

MRI Findings

Figure 3.24.1 (a–c) Axial black blood proton-density TSE images from bottom to top at three different levels demonstrate: dilatation of the right atrium (RA), with turbulent flow, and inferior vena cava (ICV), which are signs of right heart failure, hypoplastic right ventricle (RV), dilatation of the left ventricle and patent ventricular septal defect (VSD), absence of the tricuspid valve (asterisk), with fat from the atrioventricular groove interposed between the right atrium and ventricle, and Fontan conduit (FC) communicating the superior portion of the right atrium with the pulmonary artery (PA).

Figure 3.24.2 Axial balanced gradient-echo sequence shows patency of the Fontan conduit.

Figure 3.24.3 (a, b) Phase contrast images of the atriopulmonary connection and aorta and corresponding flux (ml/s) /time (ms) curves. Note the biphasic pulsatile flow in the atriopulmonary connection during the cardiac cycle, with little difference between maximal and minimal velocities. Qp/Qs was 1.5.

Further Reading

Books

Clinical Cardiac MRI. Bogaert J, *Dymarkowski* S (2005) Springer, Berlin. ISBN-13: 9783540262176

Cardiovascular Magnetic Resonance. Warren J Manning, Dudley J Pennell (2002) Churchill Livingstone, London. ISBN-13: 044307519-0

Cardiovascular MRI & MRA. Higgins Charles B, De Roos Albert (2006) Lippincott Williams & Wilkins, Philadelphia. ISBN-13: 0781762715

Cardiovascular Magnetic Resonance Imaging. Kwong Raymond Y (2008) Humana. ISBN-13: 97858829-673-3

MRI in Practice. Westbrook C, Kaut Roth C (2005) Blackwell. ISBN-13: 9781405127875

Cardiovascular Magnetic Resonance. Nagel E, van Rossum A (2004) E. Fleck. ISBN-13: 379851402x

Cardiovascular MRI. Lee VS (2006) Lippincott Williams & Wilkins. ISBN-13: 9780781779968

Cardiac Imaging, The requisites. Miller S (2004) Mosby. ISBN-13: 032301755X

Cardiovascular Imaging: A Handbook for Clinical Practice. Bax JJ, Kramer CM, Marwick TH, Wijns W (2005) Willey-Blackwell. ISBN-13: 978140513131

Novel Techniques for Imaging the Heart: Cardiac MR and CT. Di Carli MF, Kwong RY (2008) Willey-Blackwell. ISBN-13: 978140517533-3

Webs-Links

http://www.scmr.org
http://secciones.secardiologia.es/cardioRM/main.asp?w=1280
http://atlas.scmr.org/cineplayer.html
http://en.wikipedia.org/wiki/Cardiovascular_Magnetic_Resonance
http://emedicine.medscape.com/article/352250-overview
http://www.med-ed.virginia.edu/courses/rad/cardiacmr/index.html
http://www.radiologyinfo.org/en/pdf/cardiacmr.pdf
http://www.e-mri.org/cardiac-mri/introduction.html
http://www.revisemri.com/
http://www.learningradiology.com/toc/tocorgansystems/toccardiac.htm

Articles

Alfayoumi F, Gradman A, Traub D, Biedermann R. Evolving clinical application of cardiac MRI. Rev Cardiovasc Med 2007; 8:135–144

Axel L. Assessment of pericardial disease by magnetic resonance and computed tomography. J Magn Reson Imaging 2004; 19: 816–826

Abdel-Aty H, Schulz-Menger J. Cardiovascular magnetic resonance T2-weighted imaging of myocardial edema in acute myocardial infarction. Recent Pat Cardiovasc Drug Discov 2007; 2:63–68

Benza R, Biederman R, Murali S, Gupta H. Role of cardiac magnetic resonance imaging in the management of patients with pulmonary arterial hypertension. J Am Coll Cardiol 2008; 52:1683–1692

Bluemke DA, Krupinski EA, Ovitt T, Gear K, Unger E, Axel L et al MR Imaging of arrhythmogenic right ventricular cardiomyopathy: morphologic findings and interobserver reliability. Cardiology 2003; 99:153–162

Bove CM, DiMaria JM, Voros S, Conaway MR, Kramer CM. Dobutamine response and myocardial infarct transmurality: functional improvement after coronary artery bypass grafting–initial experience. Radiology 2006; 240:835–841

Buckberg G, Hoffman JI, Mahajan A, Saleh S, Coghlan C. Cardiac mechanics revisited: the relationship of cardiac architecture to ventricular function. Circulation 2008; 118:2571–2587

Carlsson M, Arheden H, Higgins CB, Saeed M. Magnetic resonance imaging as a potential gold standard for infarct quantification. J Electrocardiol 2008; 41:614–620

Chavhan GB, Babyn PS, Jankharia BG, Cheng HL, Shroff MM. Steady-state MR imaging sequences: physics, classification, and clinical applications. Radiographics 2008; 28:1147–1160

Chughtai A, Kazerooni EA. CT and MRI of acute thoracic cardiovascular emergencies. Crit Care Clin 2007; 23:835–853; vii

Constantine G, Shan K, Flamm SD, Sivananthan MU. Role of MRI in clinical cardiology. Lancet 2004; 363:2162–2171

Cook AL, Hurwitz LM, Valente AM, Herlong JR. Right heart dilatation in adults: congenital causes. AJR Am J Roentgenol 2007; 189:592–601

Crean A. Cardiovascular MR and CT in congenital heart disease. Heart 2007; 93:1637–1647

Delfino JG, Johnson KR, Eisner RL, Eder S, Leon AR, Oshinski JN. Three-directional myocardial phase-contrast tissue velocity MR imaging with navigator-echo gating: in vivo and in vitro study. Radiology 2008; 246:917–925

Dick AJ, Lederman RJ. MRI-guided myocardial cell therapy. Int J Cardiovasc Intervent 2005; 7:165–170

Dill T. Contraindications to magnetic resonance imaging: noninvasive imaging. Heart 2008; 94:943–948

Duerk JL, Wong EY, Lewin JS. A brief review of hardware for catheter tracking in magnetic resonance imaging. MAGMA 2002; 13:199–208

Festa P, Ait AL, Bernabei M, De MD. The role of magnetic resonance imaging in the evaluation of the functionally single ventricle before and after conversion to the Fontan circulation. Cardiol Young 2005; 15(Suppl 3):51–56

Finn JP, Nael K, Deshpande V, Ratib O, Laub G. Cardiac MR imaging: state of the technology. Radiology 2006; 241:338–354

gabiti-Rosei E, Muiesan ML, Salvetti M. New approaches to the assessment of left ventricular hypertrophy. Ther Adv Cardiovasc Dis 2007; 1:119–128

Gerber BL, Raman SV, Nayak K, Epstein FH, Ferreira P, Axel L et al Myocardial first-pass perfusion cardiovascular magnetic resonance: history, theory, and current state of the art. J Cardiovasc Magn Reson 2008; 10:18

Gershlick AH, de BM, Chambers J, Hackett D, Keal R, Kelion A et al Role of non-invasive imaging in the management of coronary artery disease: an assessment of likely change over the next 10 years. A report from the British Cardiovascular Society Working Group. Heart 2007; 93:423–431

Gharib AM, Elagha A, Pettigrew RI. Cardiac magnetic resonance at high field: promises and problems. Curr Probl Diagn Radiol 2008; 37:49–56

Gleeson TG, Mwangi I, Horgan SJ, Cradock A, Fitzpatrick P, Murray JG. Steady-state free-precession (SSFP) cine MRI in distinguishing normal and bicuspid aortic valves. J Magn Reson Imaging 2008; 28:873–878

Hancock EW. Differential diagnosis of restrictive cardiomyopathy and constrictive pericarditis. Heart 2001; 86:343–349

Hansen MW, Merchant N. MRI of hypertrophic cardiomyopathy: part I, MRI appearances. AJR Am J Roentgenol 2007; 189:1335–1343

Harris SR, Glockner J, Misselt AJ, Syed IS, Araoz PA. Cardiac MR imaging of nonischemic cardiomyopathies. Magn Reson Imaging Clin North Am 2008; 16:165–183; vii

Hartnell GG, Notarianni M. MRI and echocardiography: how do they compare in adults? Semin Roentgenol 1998; 33:252–261

Hauser TH, Manning WJ. The promise of whole-heart coronary MRI. Curr Cardiol Rep 2008; 10:46–50

Helm RH, Lardo AC. Cardiac magnetic resonance assessment of mechanical dyssynchrony. Curr Opin Cardiol 2008; 23: 440–446

Jerosch-Herold M, Muehling O. Stress perfusion magnetic resonance imaging of the heart. Top Magn Reson Imaging 2008; 19:33–42

Jerosch-Herold M, Kwong RY. Magnetic resonance imaging in the assessment of ventricular remodeling and viability. Curr Heart Fail Rep 2008; 5:5–10

Jeudy J, White CS. Cardiac magnetic resonance imaging: techniques and principles. Semin Roentgenol 2008; 43:173–182

Kaandorp TA, Lamb HJ, Bax JJ, van der Wall EE, de RA. Magnetic resonance imaging of coronary arteries, the ischemic cascade, and myocardial infarction. Am Heart J 2005; 149:200–208

Kaandorp TA, Lamb HJ, van der Wall EE, de RA, Bax JJ. Cardiovascular MR to access myocardial viability in chronic ischaemic LV dysfunction. Heart 2005; 91:1359–1365

Kalra MK, Abbara S. Imaging cardiac tumors. Cancer Treat Res 2008; 143:177–196

Katoh M, Stuber M, Buecker A, Gunther RW, Spuentrup E. Spin-labeling coronary MR angiography with steady-state free precession and radial k-space sampling: initial results in healthy volunteers. Radiology 2005; 236:1047–1052

Kelle S, Nagel E. Cardiovascular MRI at 3 T. Eur Radiol 2007; 17(Suppl 6):F42–F47

Kim HW, Crowley AL, Kim RJ. A clinical cardiovascular magnetic resonance service: operational considerations and the basic examination. Cardiol Clin 2007; 25:1–13; v

Knauth MA, Ordovas K, Higgins CB, Reddy GP. Magnetic resonance imaging in the adult with congenital heart disease. Semin Roentgenol 2008; 43 246–258

Kovacs G, Reiter G, Reiter U, Rienmuller R, Peacock A, Olschewski H. The emerging role of magnetic resonance imaging in the diagnosis and management of pulmonary hypertension. Respiration 2008; 76:458–470

Krishnamurthy R. Pediatric cardiac MRI: anatomy and function. Pediatr Radiol 2008; 38(Suppl 2):S192–S199

Kwong RY, Korlakunta H. Diagnostic and prognostic value of cardiac magnetic resonance imaging in assessing myocardial viability. Top Magn Reson Imaging 2008; 19:15–24

Laissy JP, Hyafil F, Feldman LJ, Juliard JM, Schouman-Claeys E, Steg PG et al Differentiating acute myocardial infarction from myocarditis: diagnostic value of early- and delayed-perfusion cardiac MR imaging. Radiology 2005; 237:75–82

Lamb HJ, van der Meer RW, de RA, Bax JJ. Cardiovascular molecular MR imaging. Eur J Nucl Med Mol Imaging 2007; 34(Suppl 1): S99–S104

Lew CD, Alley MT, Bammer R, Spielman DM, Chan FP. Peak velocity and flow quantification validation for sensitivity-encoded phase-contrast MR imaging. Acad Radiol 2007; 14:258–269

Lim RP, Srichai MB, Lee VS. Non-ischemic causes of delayed myocardial hyperenhancement on MRI. AJR Am J Roentgenol 2007; 188:1675–1681

Lin D, Kramer CM. Late gadolinium-enhanced cardiac magnetic resonance. Curr Cardiol Rep 2008; 10:72–78

Loewy J, Loewy A, Kendall EJ. Reconsideration of pacemakers and MR imaging. Radiographics 2004; 24:1257–1267

Lohan DG, Saleh R, Tomasian A, Krishnam M, Finn JP. Current status of 3-T cardiovascular magnetic resonance imaging. Top Magn Reson Imaging 2008; 19:3–13

Maceira AM, Joshi J, Prasad SK, Moon JC, Perugini E, Harding I et al Cardiovascular magnetic resonance in cardiac amyloidosis. Circulation 2005; 111:186–193

Malik TH, Bruce IA, Kaushik V, Willatt DJ, Wright NB, Rothera MP. The role of magnetic resonance imaging in the assessment of suspected extrinsic tracheobronchial compression due to vascular anomalies. Arch Dis Child 2006; 91:52–55

Marcu CB, Beek AM, van Rossum AC. Clinical applications of cardiovascular magnetic resonance imaging. CMAJ 2006; 175:911–917

Masci PG, Dymarkowski S, Bogaert J. The role of cardiovascular magnetic resonance in the diagnosis and management of cardiomyopathies. J Cardiovasc Med (Hagerstown) 2008; 9: 435–449

Masci PG, Dymarkowski S, Rademakers FE, Bogaert J. Determination of regional ejection fraction in patients with myocardial infarction by using merged late gadolinium enhancement and cine MR: feasibility study. Radiology 2009; 250:50–60

McVeigh ER, Guttman MA, Kellman P, Raval AN, Lederman RJ. Real-time, interactive MRI for cardiovascular interventions. Acad Radiol 2005; 12:1121–1127

Mertens L, Ganame J, Eyskens B. What is new in pediatric cardiac imaging? Eur J Pediatr 2008; 167:1–8

Moore P. MRI-guided congenital cardiac catheterization and intervention: the future? Catheter Cardiovasc Interv 2005; 66: 1–8

Nelson KH, Li T, Afonso L. Diagnostic approach and role of MRI in the assessment of acute myocarditis. Cardiol Rev 2009; 17: 24–30

Nieman K, Shapiro MD, Ferencik M, Nomura CH, Abbara S, Hoffmann U et al Reperfused myocardial infarction: contrast-enhanced 64-section CT in comparison to MR imaging. Radiology 2008; 247:49–56

O'Regan DP, Schmitz SA. Establishing a clinical cardiac MRI service. Clin Radiol 2006; 61:211–224

O'Sullivan PJ, Gladish GW. Cardiac tumors. Semin Roentgenol 2008; 43:223–233

Ordovas KG, Reddy GP, Higgins CB. MRI in nonischemic acquired heart disease. J Magn Reson Imaging 2008; 27: 1195–1213

Ozturk C, Guttman M, McVeigh ER, Lederman RJ. Magnetic resonance imaging-guided vascular interventions. Top Magn Reson Imaging 2005; 16:369–381

Pai VM, Axel L. Advances in MRI tagging techniques for determining regional myocardial strain. Curr Cardiol Rep 2006; 8:53–8.

Partridge JB, Anderson RH. Left ventricular anatomy: its nomenclature, segmentation, and planes of imaging. Clin Anat 2009; 22:77–84

Pennell D. Cardiovascular magnetic resonance. Heart 2001; 85: 581–589

Prasad SK, Assomull RG, Pennell DJ. Recent developments in non-invasive cardiology. BMJ 2004; 329:1386–1389

Raman VK, Lederman RJ. Interventional cardiovascular magnetic resonance imaging. Trends Cardiovasc Med 2007; 17:196–202

Ramos M, Depasquale E, Coplan NL. Assessment of myocardial viability: review of the clinical significance. Rev Cardiovasc Med 2008; 9:225–231

Reddy GP, Pujadas S, Ordovas KG, Higgins CB. MR imaging of ischemic heart disease. Magn Reson Imaging Clin North Am 2008; 16:201–12; viii

Rickers C, Wilke NM, Jerosch-Herold M, Casey SA, Panse P, Panse N et al Utility of cardiac magnetic resonance imaging in the diagnosis of hypertrophic cardiomyopathy. Circulation 2005; 112:855–861

Rodriguez E, Soler R. New MR insights of cardiomyopathy. Eur J Radiol 2008; 67:392–400

Roguin A, Schwitter J, Vahlhaus C, Lombardi M, Brugada J, Vardas P et al Magnetic resonance imaging in individuals with cardiovascular implantable electronic devices. Europace 2008; 10:336–346

Sa MI, de RA, Westenberg JJ, Kroft LJ. Imaging techniques in cardiac resynchronization therapy. Int J Cardiovasc Imaging 2008; 24:89–105

Sahn DJ, Vick GW III. Review of new techniques in echocardiography and magnetic resonance imaging as applied to patients with congenital heart disease. Heart 2001; 86(Suppl 2): II41–II53

Sakuma H, Higgins CB. Magnetic resonance measurement of coronary blood flow. Acta Paediatr Suppl 2004; 93:80–85

Salanitri J, Lisle D, Rigsby C, Slaughter R, Edelman R. Benign cardiac tumours: cardiac CT and MRI imaging appearances. J Med Imaging Radiat Oncol 2008; 52:550–558

Sarwar A, Shapiro MD, Abbara S, Cury RC. Cardiac magnetic resonance imaging for the evaluation of ventricular function. Semin Roentgenol 2008; 43:183–192

Saxena SK, Sharma M, Patel M, Oreopoulos D. Nephrogenic systemic fibrosis: an emerging entity. Int Urol Nephrol 2008; 40: 715–724

Scott AD, Keegan J, Firmin DN. Motion in cardiovascular MR imaging. Radiology 2009; 250:331–351

Sen-Chowdhry S, McKenna WJ. The utility of magnetic resonance imaging in the evaluation of arrhythmogenic right ventricular cardiomyopathy. Curr Opin Cardiol 2008; 23: 38–45

Sena L. Cardiac MR imaging: from physics to protocols. Pediatr Radiol 2008; 38(Suppl 2):S185–S191

Shapiro MD, Guarraia DL, Moloo J, Cury RC. Evaluation of acute coronary syndromes by cardiac magnetic resonance imaging. Top Magn Reson Imaging 2008; 19:25–32

Shehata ML, Turkbey EB, Vogel-Claussen J, Bluemke DA. Role of cardiac magnetic resonance imaging in assessment of nonischemic cardiomyopathies. Top Magn Reson Imaging 2008; 19:43–57

Shinbane JS, Colletti PM, Shellock FG. MR in patients with pacemakers and ICDs: defining the issues. J Cardiovasc Magn Reson 2007; 9:5–13

Sklansky M. Advances in fetal cardiac imaging. Pediatr Cardiol 2004; 25:307–321

Slomka PJ, Berman DS, Germano G. Applications and software techniques for integrated cardiac multimodality imaging. Expert Rev Cardiovasc Ther 2008; 6:27–41

Sparrow PJ, Kurian JB, Jones TR, Sivananthan MU. MR imaging of cardiac tumors. Radiographics 2005; 25:1255–1276

Steel KE, Kwong RY. Application of cardiac magnetic resonance imaging in cardiomyopathy. Curr Heart Fail Rep 2008; 5:128–135

Strach K, Meyer C, Schild H, Sommer T. Cardiac stress MR imaging with dobutamine. Eur Radiol 2006; 16:2728–2738

Strzelczyk J, Attili A. Cardiac magnetic resonance evaluation of myocardial viability and ischemia. Semin Roentgenol 2008; 43:193–203

Taylor AM. Cardiac imaging: MR or CT? Which to use when. Pediatr Radiol 2008; 38(Suppl 3):S433–S438

Tomlinson DR, Becher H, Selvanayagam JB. Assessment of myocardial viability: comparison of echocardiography versus cardiac magnetic resonance imaging in the current era. Heart Lung Circ 2008; 17:173–185

van der Geest RJ, Lelieveldt BP, Reiber JH. Quantification of global and regional ventricular function in cardiac magnetic resonance imaging. Top Magn Reson Imaging 2000; 11:348–358

Varghese A, Keegan J, Pennell DJ. Cardiovascular magnetic resonance of anomalous coronary arteries. Coron Artery Dis 2005; 16:355–364

Weaver JC, McCrohon JA. Contrast-enhanced cardiac MRI in myocardial infarction. Heart Lung Circ 2008; 17:290–298

Weinsaft JW, Klem I, Judd RM. MRI for the assessment of myocardial viability. Cardiol Clin 2007; 25:35–56; v

White JA, Patel MR. The role of cardiovascular MRI in heart failure and the cardiomyopathies. Cardiol Clin 2007; 25:71–95; vi

Wieben O, Francois C, Reeder SB. Cardiac MRI of ischemic heart disease at 3 T: potential and challenges. Eur J Radiol 2008; 65: 15–28

Nuclear Cardiology

José Manuel Jiménez-Hoyuela García

Simeón Ortega Lozano, Dolores Martínez del Valle Torres,
Antonio Guitiérrez Cardo, and Esperanza Ramos Moreno (Contributors)

Introduction

Heart disease is the leading cause of death in developed countries, as well as in many developing countries. The prevalence of heart disease is increasing with increasing life expectancy and gains in socioeconomic conditions. In many patients with no clinical history suggestive of heart problems, heart disease strikes unexpectedly in the form of myocardial infarction or sudden death. Therefore, apart from its efforts to prevent heart disease by controlling risk factors, the medical community has strived to improve the early detection of heart disease, especially of the asymptomatic form or "silent ischemia," to avert its potential consequences.

Nuclear cardiology tests to study myocardial perfusion and ventricular function have developed into indispensable tools for the diagnosis and evaluation of heart disease.

Heart disease is caused by arteriosclerosis in the epicardial vessels; this systemic disorder of metabolic origin causes progressive narrowing of sections of the vascular lumen. Even in cases with severe stenoses in which the vascular lumen is reduced by 80 or 90%, coronary blood flow seems sufficient to enable functional contractility when the patient is at rest; however, when metabolic demand increases, less severe stenoses can cause ischemia due to the disequilibrium between the supply and the demand of oxygen.

The usual sequence of events known as the "ischemic cascade" begins with a regional alteration in myocardial perfusion; metabolic changes follow and lead to contractile dysfunction and electrocardiographic modifications that culminate in clinical signs like angor. In any case, altered perfusion is considered the main factor conditioning the ischemia, but altered perfusion is difficult to demonstrate in baseline conditions, even using invasive methods. For this reason, increased coronary blood flow is the basis for demonstrating heterogeneous myocardial perfusion that reflects regional decreases in the coronary reserve in response to a direct or indirect vasodilating stimulus, whether physiological (exercise) or pharmacological (vasoactive or inotropic drugs).

Single photon emission computed tomography (SPECT) analyzes the distribution of radionuclide in the myocardium in tomographic images in three axes; the different ventricular walls are analyzed in each axis and correlations are established with the distribution of irrigation from the coronary arteries. In recent years, the possibility of obtaining perfusion images in synchronization with the electrocardiogram, or ECG-gated SPECT, enables us to study two key aspects in the diagnosis and prognosis of heart disease – myocardial perfusion and ventricular function – in the same examination. ECG gating has improved the diagnostic accuracy of myocardial perfusion studies and increased their specificity by enabling better identification of attenuation artefacts and better assessment of the severity of ischemic heart disease.

All these circumstances make nuclear cardiology and especially myocardial perfusion studies an efficacious noninvasive method for the diagnostic and prognostic evaluation of heart disease.

Case 4.1

Left Bundle-Branch Block (LBBB)

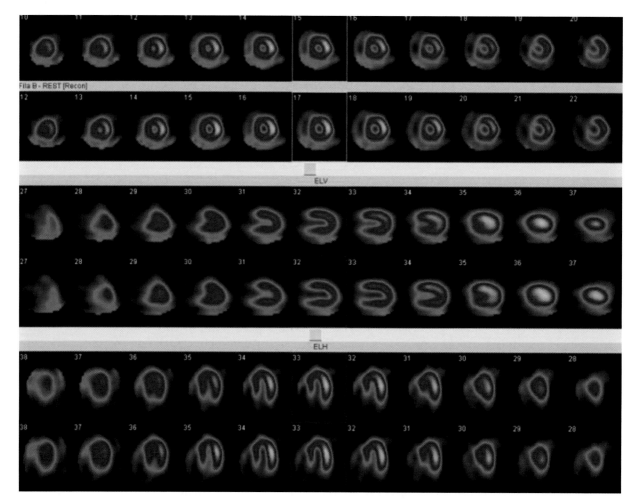

Fila B - REST [Recon]

Fig. 4.1.1

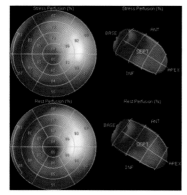

Fig. 4.1.2

Fig. 4.1.3

A 54-year-old man consulted for oppressive chest pain. He was a heavy smoker and had various episodes of typical angina, which had become more frequent in the month prior to consultation. The ECG showed left bundle branch block.

Coronary artery disease was suspected and he was referred for radionuclide myocardial perfusion imaging. A 2-day Tc-99m-tetrofosmin protocol was used. The stress test was carried out using pharmacologically induced coronary hyperemia (adenosine i.v., 140 mg/kg/min, 6 min). Coronary angiography was normal.

Comments

Because LBBB renders ECG stress testing nondiagnostic, a noninvasive diagnosis of coronary artery disease (CAD) is often sought by using radionuclide myocardial perfusion imaging.

LBBB causes septal wall motion abnormalities and reduces systolic septal wall thickness. Patients with LBBB may demonstrate septal or anteroseptal perfusion abnormalities in the absence of demonstrable CAD.

Reversible and fixed false-positive septal defects are observed in LBBB. Transient septal defects occur during exercise perfusion imaging in the absence of left anterior descending coronary artery disease in 20–50% of patients with LBBB. Several mechanisms have been proposed to explain perfusion defects. Diminished septal perfusion at exercise due to asynchronous septal relaxation that is out of phase with diastolic coronary filling has been proposed. Other mechanisms proposed include prolonged compression of septal perforators, reduced diastolic flow, small vessel CAD, septal fibrosis, and wall motion artifacts.

In general, pharmacological stress scintigraphy should routinely be used instead of conventional exercise scintigraphy in patients with LBBB and chest pain of suspected ischemic origin.

Imaging Findings

Figure 4.1.1 Short axis, vertical long axis, and horizontal long axis stress and rest images are shown in the first *two rows*. Stress/rest perfusion imaging demonstrates a nonreversible septal defect. False-positive image caused by left bundle branch block (LBBB).

Figure 4.1.2 Quantitative polar plots measuring regional myocardial perfusion show a fixed septal defect caused by LBBB.

Figure 4.1.3 Quantitative polar plots measuring regional myocardial wall motion and wall thickening from gated-SPECT demonstrate dyskinesia–hypokinesia in the septal region caused by LBBB.

Case 4.2
■
Breast Attenuation

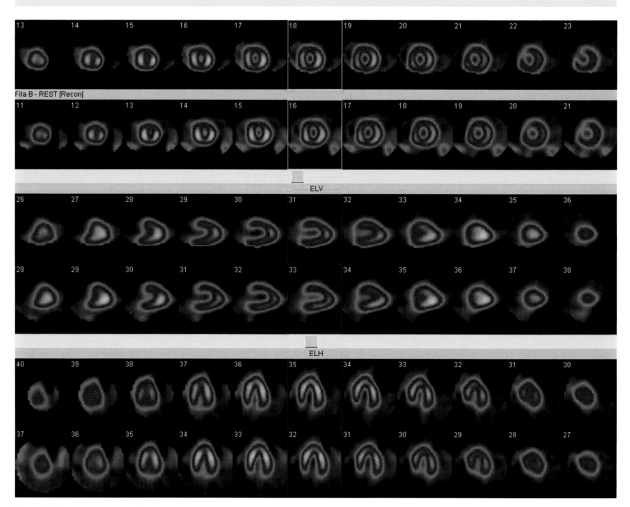

Fig. 4.2.1

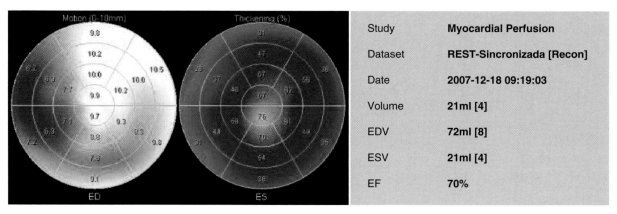

Study	**Myocardial Perfusion**
Dataset	**REST-Sincronizada [Recon]**
Date	**2007-12-18 09:19:03**
Volume	**21ml [4]**
EDV	**72ml [8]**
ESV	**21ml [4]**
EF	**70%**

Fig. 4.2.2

A hypertensive 78-year-old female exsmoker presented with oppressive nonradiating chest pain on moderate exercise, suggesting angina on exercise.

Breast attenuation causes a pseudo-defect of uptake in the anterior region, apex, or lateral side, depending on the size and the position of the breast. These defects are generally permanent and are not easily confused with ischemia. However, they can occasionally be confused with nontransmural necrosis without associated perilesional ischemia. In these cases, it is essential to evaluate the morphology and location of the defect. It is also important to thoroughly evaluate regional wall motion and wall thickening using GATED-SPECT.

Myocardial perfusion single-proton emission computed tomography (SPECT) is done with TC99m-Tetrofosmin over 2 days and the study is synchronized with the R wave (gated-SPECT) during rest and during pharmacologically induced stress.

Figure 4.2.1 Slightly reduced uptake in the anterior territory is observed, with no significant changes at rest.

Figure 4.2.2 In the synchronized study (gated-SPECT), no significant findings were observed, yet wall motion alterations were appreciated. Normal ventricular volumes and ejection fraction were found. The alterations in anterior uptake are produced by breast attenuation.

Case 4.3
■
Diaphragmatic Attenuation

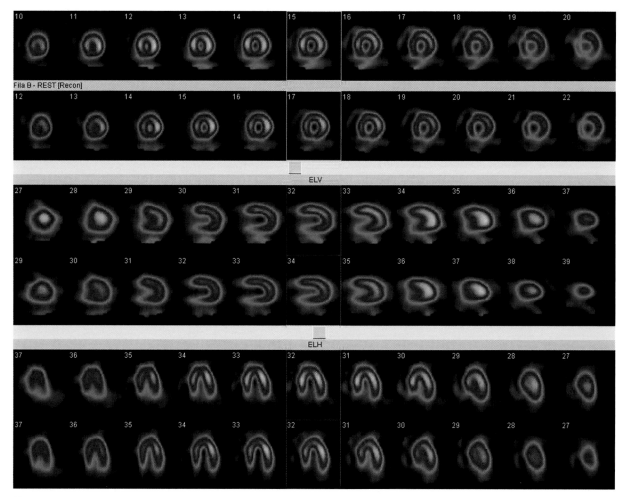

Fig. 4.3.1

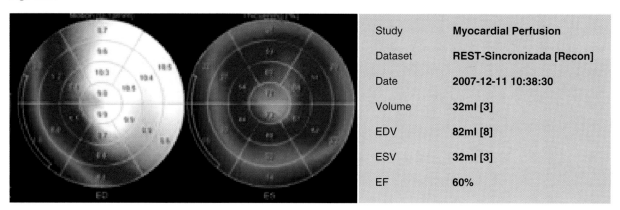

Study	**Myocardial Perfusion**
Dataset	**REST-Sincronizada [Recon]**
Date	**2007-12-11 10:38:30**
Volume	**32ml [3]**
EDV	**82ml [8]**
ESV	**32ml [3]**
EF	**60%**

Fig. 4.3.2

An obese, hypertensive, 65-year-old male smoker presented with a clinical history of chest pain and angina on exertion.

Diaphragmatic attenuation is common in males, probably due to a larger, more muscular diaphragm. Attenuation depends on the patient's size, shape, and anatomy. It can be so intense that it causes a defect in the inferior wall. These defects are fixed, and in general are not confused with ischemia, but they can be mistaken for areas of necrosis. To differentiate diaphragmatic attentuation from nontransmural necrosis without associated ischemia, appearance and location (in general, attenuations are usually more basal) must be considered with the help of the R-wave synchronized study (gated-SPECT), which is usually normal with no evidence of alterations in wall motion in these patients.

Myocardial perfusion imaging is performed with Tc99m-Tetrofosmin over 2 days and includes an R-wave synchronized study (gated-SPECT) during pharmacologically induced stress.

Figure 4.3.1 No significant defects in the distribution of the myocardial outline are shown. Only one area of slightly reduced uptake is shown in the inferior side, with minimal extension and intensity.

Figure 4.3.2 In the R-wave synchronized study (gated-SPECT), no significant findings are shown; wall motion and systolic thickening are preserved. Ventricular volumes are normal. There are no significant defects; the area of reduced uptake is compatible with diaphragmatic physiological attenuation.

Case 4.4
■
Inducible Ischemia in the CX Territory

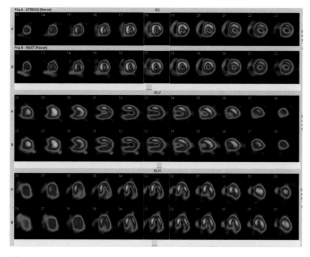

Fig. 4.4.1

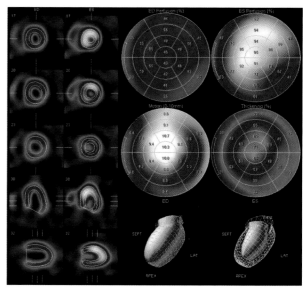

Fig. 4.4.3

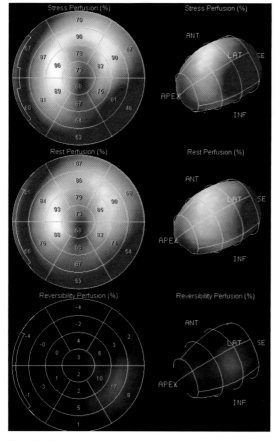

Fig. 4.4.2

A 66-year-old man with a history of arterial hypertension and no other cardiovascular risk factors presented with oppressive chest pain on moderate exercise of 3 months' evolution. The baseline electrocardiogram showed no significant alterations.

Myocardial perfusion SPECT using Tc99m tetrofosmin (925 Mbq (25 mCi)) was carried out over 2 days and included an exercise stress study and a rest study. The Bruce protocol was used for the treadmill test, with the patient exercising for 4 min and 49 s, reaching 70% of the anticipated maximum heart frequency, and 6.00 METs; the test finished when the patient was exhausted. The test was clinically and electrically negative.

Myocardial perfusion images were acquired in synchronization with the R wave (gated-SPECT).

Comments

Although myocardial perfusion images are less sensitive when the level reached is lower than what is considered adequate (1), the results observed in this case show the existence of inclusive inducible ischemia when the stress test has been below optimal conditions.

According to the polar maps that quantify the findings, the perfusion defect is theoretically due to a lesion in the circumflex coronary artery. However, wide ranges of overlapping between the territories supplied by the circumflex coronary artery and the right coronary artery have been observed (2).

Perfusion studies are superior to other noninvasive methods in the diagnosis of single-vessel disease (3), and alterations detected in the lateral side are particularly interesting. Several studies have shown the specificity of defects associated to the circumflex coronary artery in the diagnosis of ischemic heart disease on myocardial perfusion SPECT images. It is more difficult to evaluate the circumflex coronary artery territory due to the existence of other simultaneous lesions (4).

Imaging Findings

Figures 4.4.1 and 4.4.2 Moderately reduced uptake is observed in the inferolateral territory at the level of the medial and basal segments in the post-stress study. The images obtained at rest demonstrate complete reversibility in the areas affected at stress.

Figure 4.4.3 The study synchronized with the R wave through QGS shows inferolateral hypokinesia and normal ventricular volumes: End-diastolic volume: 82 ml, end-systolic volume: 36 ml, ejection fraction: 55%.

The findings are compatible with inducible ischemia in the theoretical territory of the circumflex coronary artery.

Case 4.5
■
Infarct with Residual Ischemia

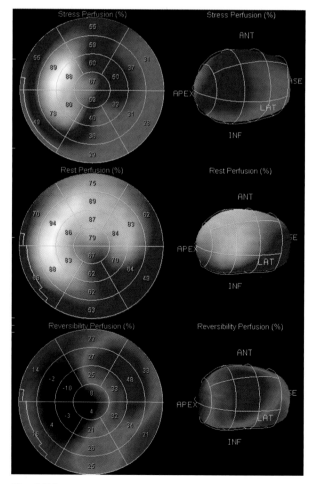

Fig. 4.5.1

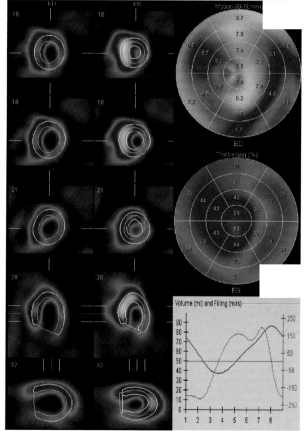

Fig. 4.5.2

A hypertensive 58-year-old man with dyslipemia and a history of inferoposterior myocardial infarction and reinfarction the following year presented with functional class II stable chronic angina and early positive treadmill exercise test (three-vessel disease with occlusion of arched and of the right coronary artery).

The patient underwent myocardial perfusion SPECT for persistent angina with early positive stress test.

Comments

The diagnostic value of myocardial perfusion imaging after an infarct comes from the evaluation of the residual ischemia in the infarcted territory as well as in other territories through the ischemia test and from the demonstration of ventricular dysfunction. These two factors are the principle physiopathological mechanisms that determine the diagnosis and evolution of the infarct during the first year and after 5 years.

Partially reversible defects are interpreted as areas in which ischemic and scarred myocardial tissue coexist (infarct zone).

The criteria for evaluating the defect can vary according to the sensitivity and specificity required.

The reversibility of the myocardial uptake in the region of the infarct suggests residual ischemia at this level, which can be due to permeability of the artery related to the infarct and/or to the existence of collateral circulation.

An objective way to quantify the extension of the necrosis and the residual ischemia is through polar maps (see image). The extension of the necrosis will be represented by any uptake inferior to 40% with respect to the maximum at rest. The zone of perilesional ischemia will be defined by a difference >10% in uptake in the infarcted zone between the rest test and the stress test.

The mortality rate of patients that have suffered a myocardial infarct without complications during the acute phase is usually between 1 and 5%. It is important to define patients at "low risk," those with negative study who should receive conservative treatment, as opposed to those at "high risk," who have ischemia. The latter group includes those who can benefit from coronary revascularization, as well as so-called nonrevascularizable patients, who are treated through cardiac rehabilitation (as in this case).

Findings

Figure 4.5.1 Inferolateral wall infarct together with lateral and inferior ischemia. Polar and quantitative images of the volume show reversibility of ischemia for the lateral and inferior sides.

Figure 4.5.2 The R-wave synchronized study shows evident post-stress dilatation, hypokinesia, and enlargement of reduced uptake areas and worsening of ventricular function that recuperated at rest, together with persistent basal inferolateral hypokinesia.

These findings indicate severe inducible ischemia by stress in the lateral and inferior sides and basal inferolateral necrosis.

Case 4.6

■

Ischemia in the Ada Territory

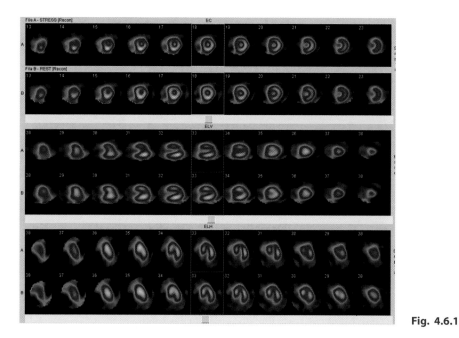

Fig. 4.6.1

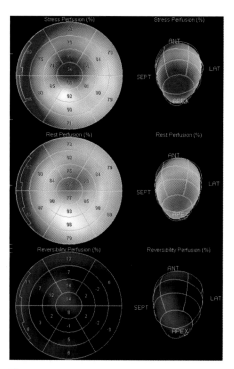

Fig. 4.6.2

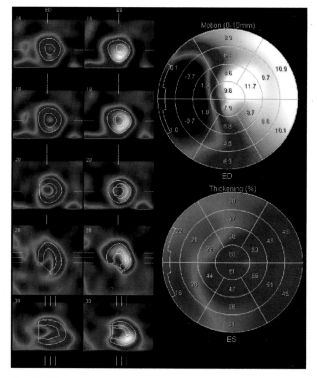

Fig. 4.6.3

A 75-year-old woman with a history of type-2 diabetes mellitus, arterial hypertension, hypercholesterolemia, obesity, degenerative arthritis, knee replacement surgery, circulatory insufficiency, and paroxysmal supraventricular tachycardia with frequent crises of intranodal tachycardia treated with ablation 7 years prior presented with episodes of chest pain with electric changes and was diagnosed with ischemic heart disease.

Myocardial perfusion SPECT imaging synchronized with the R wave (gated-SPECT) was performed over 2 days. Stress was pharmacologically induced (0.160 mg/min adenosine for 6 min) and another study was performed at rest. No incidents were observed during stress induction.

Comments

The findings described show concentric hypertrophy of the left ventricular and diastolic dysfunction related to the history of arterial hypertension, which is the most frequent cause of left ventricular hypertrophy.

In patients with a small ventricular cavity, more frequent in females, and left ventricular hypertrophy, it is more difficult to detect the endocardial border accurately and it is easy to underestimate the end-systolic volume; accurate detection of the endocardial border and correct measurement of end-systolic volume are important for the correct interpretation of the result of the gated-SPECT study.

Reduced uptake in the anterior territory can be confused with breast attenuation but the changes noted show the existence of ischemia inducible by pharmacological stress, with a mild extension and moderate intensity in the territory corresponding to the anterior descending artery.

The patient presented multiple cardiovascular risk factors and it was impossible to carry out a conventional stress test. In this type of patients, myocardial perfusion imaging with pharmacologically induced stress enables inducible ischemia to be detected with great success.

Imaging Findings

Figures 4.6.1 and 4.6.2 The post-stress study shows reduced apical and anteroapical uptake with complete reversibility in the rest study.

Figure 4.6.3 The R-wave synchronized study shows anomalous septal wall motion, without significant alterations. The volume curve is compatible with diastolic dysfunction.

Case 4.7

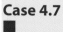

Ischemia in the Right Coronary Artery Territory

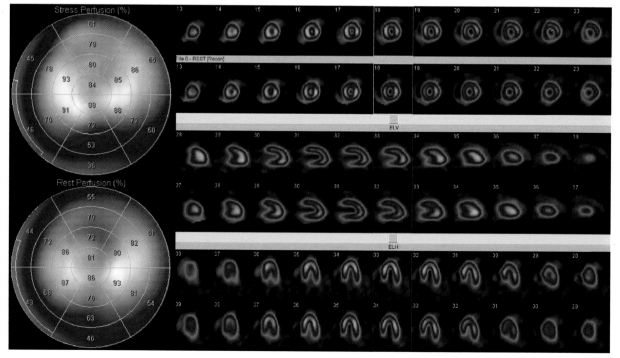

Fig. 4.7.1

A 51-year-old man with history of diabetes mellitus treated with oral antidiabetics, high blood pressure, and smoking presented with typical angina. No pathological findings were observed at EKG, and no significant alterations were found at echocardiography. A submaximal treadmill exercise test was clinically and electrically negative.

Given his typical chest pain and cardiovascular risk factors, a myocardial perfusion study was requested to rule out inducible ischemia.

Comments

Myocardial perfusion studies with tomographic acquisition are superior to other noninvasive techniques for diagnosing the status of single-vessel disease. Single-vessel lesions that go undiagnosed are usually severe stenosis (<90%). The diagnosis is more or less accurate depending on the affected vessels, with acceptable results for the anterior descending artery and the right coronary artery (RCA). In this case (RCA), the sensitivity obtained is around 75% with a slightly higher specificity (85%).

Findings

Figure 4.7.1 In the images obtained after the treadmill exercise stress test, reduced uptake is seen in the inferior territory and in the inferolateral area at the level of the medium and posterior segments, which show changes in the rest study. The R-wave synchronized study (gated-SPECT) did not show any significant alterations and ventricular volumes and EF were normal. These findings suggest the existence of inducible ischemia in the hypothetical territory of the RCA.

Case 4.8

■

Infarct in the Apex and Anteroinferior Apical Segments Without Residual Ischemia. Inducible Ischemia in the Inferolateral Side

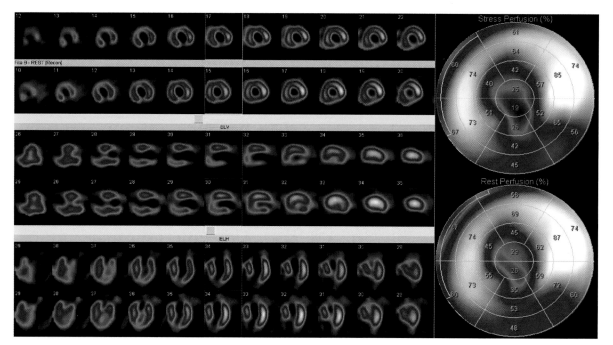

Fig. 4.8.1

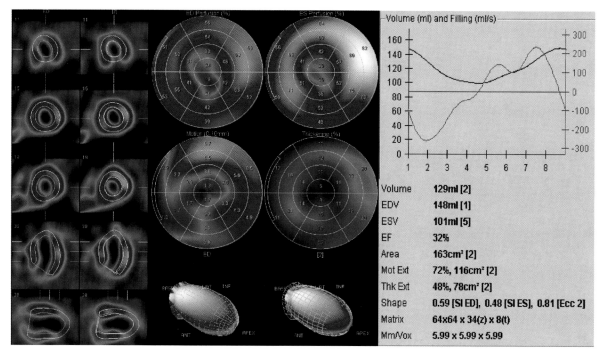

Fig. 4.8.2

A 70-year-old man presented with chest pain of short duration that irradiated to the back occurring almost daily. He had a history of an extensive ischemic-type infarct 3 years prior treated with stenting of the anterior descending coronary artery.

Myocardial perfusion defects can be classified by their scintigraphic behavior and the intensity of uptake in ischemic lesions or infarcted areas. The primary xxx are those which present "cold defects" or reduced uptake in the stress test that disappears in the basal study (see lateral and inferior territory in image x). In cases of infarct, the uptake defect remains stable in both studies.

Moderate or severe defects that remain unchanged in the at-rest study are called "fixed defects." Fixed defects usually correspond to an infarct with a higher or lower degree of transmutability, although less frequently, they have also been found to be related with areas of fibrosis.

Myocardial perfusion images enable the size of the infarcted area to be evaluated. There is a good correlation between the extension of the myocardium with reduced uptake and the degree of alteration in the segmented contractility and the ejection fraction at rest.

The values of global and regional systolic function bring significant added value to the analysis of tomographic images acquired during stress and at rest.

These examinations are cost-efficient and enable the contractility analysis of regional wall motion and wall thickening. The most relevant variables in cardiologic patients are the location of ischemia, ejection fraction (EF), ventricular volumes, and evaluation of regional myocardial viability.

The EF of the left ventricle is considered the most important prognostic variable after an acute myocardial infarct, although few patients have low EF (<40%). Gated-SPECT assesses the degree of systolic dysfunction of the left ventricle; a decrease in EF greater than 5% with respect to the baseline during stress predicts future ischemic events.

Transitory ventricular dilatation is typical of patients with severe coronary artery disease in whom a high volume of EF with decreased ventricular function is produced during the stress test.

Figure 4.8.1 Tomographic study with myocardial perfusion images through dynamic exercise stress (BRUCE protocol): the perfusion images show absence of uptake (cold defect) in the apex and antero- and infero-apical segments that do not demonstrate reversibility in the rest study. There is reduced uptake in the inferior and inferolateral territories with changes in the medial and inferior segments.

Figure 4.8.2 Results of the QGS: on the left, the selected images in diastole and systole. Above on the right, the perfusion polar maps followed by the wall motion polar maps (global hypokinesia with apical dyskinetic movement) and systolic thickening. Below, the images of the epicardium appear as a wire mesh and the endocardium as a shaded surface in the lateral oblique projection. Volume curve obtained: ventricular dysfunction pattern. High ventricular volumes and depressed EF.

Case 4.9
■
Multivessel Disease

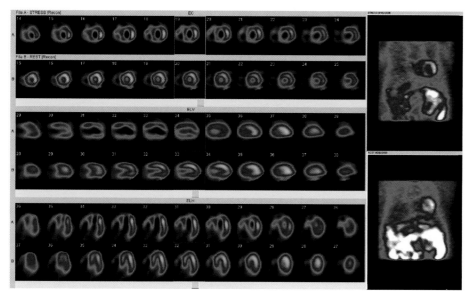

Fig. 4.9.1

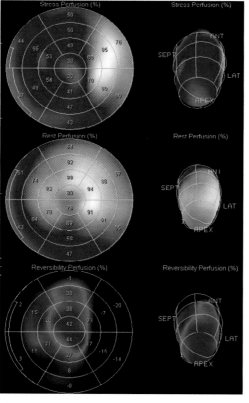

Fig. 4.9.2

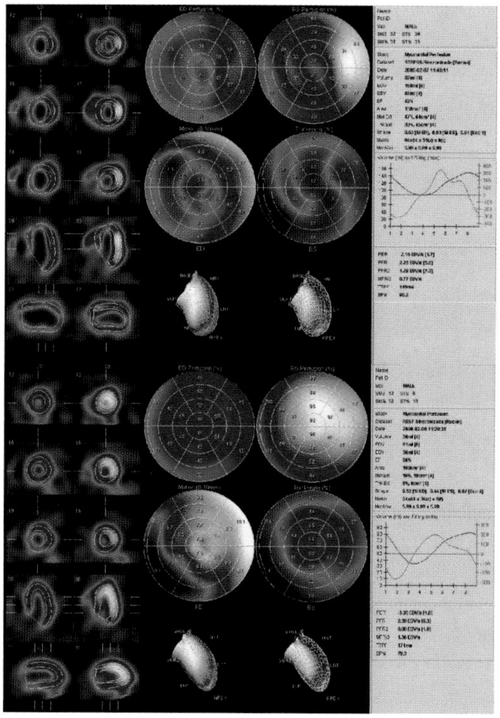

Fig. 4.9.3

A 66-year-old man with a history of type-2 diabetes mellitus, arterial hypertension, and smoking presented with chest pain on stress suggestive of angina over the previous 6 months; he had no pain at rest. The findings at physical examination were normal. The EKG showed sinus rhythm with right bundle branch block. Chest X-ray and blood tests were normal except hyperglycemia. He was diagnosed with functional class II angina on exertion.

Myocardial perfusion SPECT using tetrofosmine-Tc99m 925 Mbq (25mCi) was carried out with treadmill exercise stress testing and at rest testing over 2 days. The Bruce protocol was used for the treadmill exercise stress test, with exercise lasting 4 min and 45 s and reaching 99% of the expected maximum heart rate, 3 MET. The test was negative; electrical data were not useful due to right bundle brunch block.

The myocardial SPECT (myocardial perfusion imaging) study was completed through R-wave synchronized (gated-SPECT) imaging.

Findings

Figures 4.9.1 and 4.9.2 Increased lung uptake was observed in the post-stress study. An extensive area of moderately reduced uptake was observed in the anterior, septal, inferolateral, and apical areas. The at-rest study showed complete reversibility of the uptake defects in these areas.

Figure 4.9.3 The evaluation of the R-wave synchronized study through quantitative gated-SPECT (QGS) after stress showed global hypokinesia. No alterations were observed in the at-rest study.

Ventricular volumes and ejection fraction after stress were end-diastolic volume: 150 ml; end-systolic volume: 87 ml; EF: 42%. After rest: end-diastolic volume: 81 ml; end-systolic volume: 36 ml; EF: 56%.

Comments

The findings described are compatible with inducible ischemia in the theoretical territory of the right coronary and anterior descending arteries with certain scintigraphic severity and stunned myocardium in the post-stress study. The criteria for severity are extensive ischemia, intense ischemia, augmented lung uptake in stress, ischemic dilatation of the left ventricle, and decreased post-stress ventricular function.

Technetium tracers are less sensitive than thallium in detecting pulmonary activity, but elevated lung uptake is also an indicator of the severity of coronary disease and of ventricular dysfunction.

In cases of severe coronary disease, transitory dilatation with associated ventricular dysfunction is seen in the SPECT images. This finding is more frequently observed in studies using thallium-201 and fast image acquisition. In studies using technetium tracers, this finding may also be present in cases of diffuse coronary disease.

The existence of multivessel disease increases the sensitivity of gated-SPECT myocardial perfusion studies.

Case 4.10

■

Stunned Myocardium

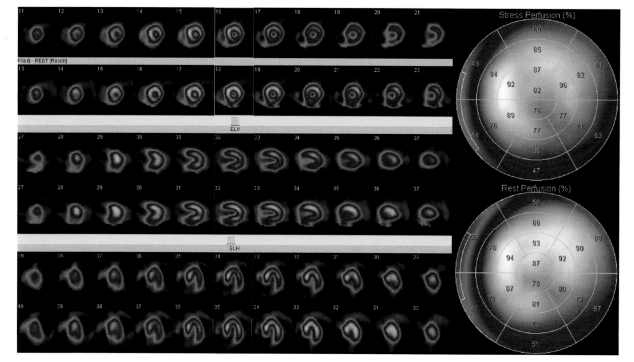

Fig. 4.10.1

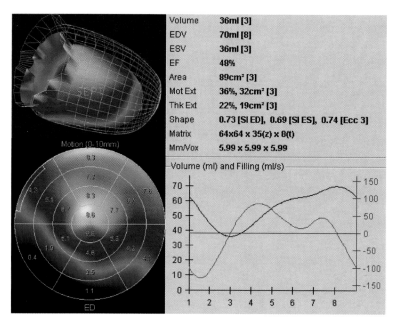

Volume	36ml [3]
EDV	70ml [8]
ESV	36ml [3]
EF	48%
Area	89cm² [3]
Mot Ext	36%, 32cm² [3]
Thk Ext	22%, 19cm² [3]
Shape	0.73 [SI ED], 0.69 [SI ES], 0.74 [Ecc 3]
Matrix	64x64 x 35(z) x 8(t)
Mm/Vox	5.99 x 5.99 x 5.99

Fig. 4.10.2

A 78-year-old man was sent to our department for the evaluation of possible residual ischemia after myocardial infarction and fibrinolysis 1 week before. The patient was stabilized and had no symptoms of angina.

Myocardial perfusion study was carried out with pharmacological stress and R-wave synchronized study (gated-SPECT).

Comments

The concept of myocardial stunning was first described in 1975 by Vatner. Later, Braunwald and Kloner named this phenomenon "myocardial stunning" to refer to a reversible form of contractile dysfunction that can occur after restoration of coronary blood flow following a relatively brief period of coronary occlusion. This damage conditioned by reperfusion has been related, among other factors, with the sudden readministration of calcium and oxygen, with the generation of free radicals, with mitochondria dysfunction, with the infiltration of several inflammatory cells, and with the generation of multiple humoral factors causing the inflammation. From the clinical point of view, myocardial stunning can cause morbimortality. Other aspects must also be considered; for instance, the ejection fraction (a very important factor for the prognosis) resulting from myocardial stunning is not real and can be more or less underestimated depending on the degree of shock. Contractility cannot be used to evaluate viability in a postischemic myocardium and repetitive episodes of shock can lead to chronic alterations.

Findings

Figure 4.10.1 No significant defects were found in the myocardial perfusion study after pharmacological stress.

Figure 4.10.2 The R-wave synchronized study showed marked hypokinesia in the inferior territory with akinesia at the level of the inferoposterior segment. Ventricular volumes were slightly elevated with a slight decrease in the ejection fraction of the left ventricle. This is, therefore, a case of acute coronary occlusion that was effectively treated leading to reperfusion that prevented myocardial infarction, although myocardial stunning occurred in the inferior side.

Further Reading

Books

Ortega Alcalde D, Pereztol Valdés O. Radiofármacos, adquisición y procesamiento. In: Candell J, Castell J, Aguadé S (ed) Cardiología nuclear en la práctica clínica. Aula Médica, Madrid, 2003; 47–88

Nichols KJ, Galt JR. Quality control for SPECT imaging. In: De Puey EG, Berman DS, García EV (edrs) Cardiac SPECT Imaging. Raven, New York, 1995; 24–47

Diagnostic Nuclear Medicine. Sandler MP, Coleman MP, Paton JA, Wackers FJ, Gottschalk A (2004) Lippincott Williams & Wilkins, Philadelphia

Nuclear Cardiology, Practical Applications. Heller GV, Hendel RC (2004) McGraw Hill, New York

Castell Conesa J, Aguadé Bruix S. Estudios de perfusión miocárdica. In: Candell J, Castell J, Aguadé S (eds) Cardiología nuclear en la práctica clínica. Aula Médica, Madrid, 2003; 47–88

Avances tecnológicos en el SPECT de perfusión miocárdica. En Castro-Beiras JM Ernest V García, César A. Santana, Tracy L. Faber (2004) Meditecnica, Madrid, 71–83

Castell J, Cortadellas A. Criterios de interpretación del SPECT. In: Candell J, Castell J, Aguadé S (eds) Miocardio en riesgo y miocardio viable. Diagnóstico mediante SPECT. Barcelona, Doyma, 1998; 29–50

Rizvi A, Velusamy M, Helder G. Evaluation of myocardial viability. In: Heller G, Hendel R (eds) Nuclear Cardiology Practical Applications. McGraw-Hill, New York, 2004; 49–66

Web-links

www.asnc.org

http://brighamrad.harvard.edu/education/online/Cardiac/Cardiac.html/

www.acc.org

http://www.bncs.org.uk/

http://journals.elsevierhealth.com/periodicals/ymnc

http://www.nucmedinfo.com/Pages/nuccardiologybase.html

www.escardio.org

www.semn.es

www.ecnc.nuclearcardiology.org

www.britishcardiacresearch.org

Articles

Fundamentals

Brindis RG, Douglas PS, Hendel RC, Peterson ED, Wolk MJ, Allen JM, et al ACCF/ASNC Appropriateness criteria for Single-Photon Emission Computed Tomography Myocardial Perfusion Imaging (SPECT MPI). A report of the American College of Cardiology Foundation Quality Strategic Directions Committee Appropriateness Criteria Working Group and the American Society of Nuclear Cardiology. J Am Coll Cardiol 2005; 46:1587–1605

Dahlberg ST, Leppo JA. Myocardial kinetics of radiolabeled perfusion agents: basis for perfusion imaging. J Nucl Cardiol 1994; 1:189–197

Hesse B, Tägil K, Cuocolo A, Anagnostopoulos C, Bardiés M, Bax J et al EANM/ESC procedural gudelines for myocardial perfusion imaging in nuclear cardiology. Eur J Nucl Med Mol Imaging 2005; 32:855–897

Klocke FJ, Baird MG, Lorell BH, Bateman TM, Messer JV, Berman DS et al ACC/AHA/ASNC guidelines for the clinical use of cardiac radionuclide imaging: executive summary. A report of the American College of Cardiology/American Heart Association Task Force on Practice Guidelines (ACC/AHA/ASNC Committee to revise the 1995 Guidelines for the clinical use of cardiac radionuclide imaging). Circulation 2003; 108:1404–1018

Normal Patient

Diagnostic Nuclear Medicine. Sandler MP, Coleman MP, Paton JA, Wackers FJ, Gottschalk A (2004) Lippincott Williams & Wilkins, Philadelphia

Nuclear Cardiology, Practical Applications. Heller GV, Hendel RC (2004) McGraw Hill, New York

Cerqueira M. Nuclear cardiology: finally a one-stop shop for diagnosis, risk stratification, and management of coronary artery disease. Clin Cardiol 2006; 29(9):126–133

Kontos MC, Tatum JL. Imaging in the evaluation of the patient with suspected acute coronary syndrome. Semin Nucl Med 2003; 33(4):246–258

Metz LD, Beattie M, Hom R, Redberg RF, Grady D, Fleischmann KE. The prognostic value of normal exercise myocardial perfusion imaging and exercise echocardiography: a meta-analysis. J Am Coll Cardiol 2007; 16(49):227–237

Russell RR III, Zaret B. Nuclear cardiology: present and future. Curr Probl Cardiol 2006; 31(9):557–629

Breast Attenuation

Hamsen CL, Sundaram S. The ratio of the apex/anterior wall: marker of breast attenuation artifact in women. Nucl Med Commun 2006; 27(10):803–806

Movahed MR. Attenuation artifact during myocardial SPECT imaging secondary to saline and silicone breast implants. Am Heart Hosp J 2007; 5(3):195–196

Santana C, Candel J, Castell J, Aguadé S, García A, Canela T, González JM, Cortadellas J, Ortega D, Soler J. Diagnostic accuracy of technetium-99m- MIBI myocardial SPECT in women and men. J Nucl Med 1998; 39:751–755

Diaphragmatic Attenuation

Hamsen CL, Sundaram S. The ratio of the apex/anterior wall: marker of breast attenuation artifact in women. Nucl Med Commun 2006; 27(10)803–806

Movahed MR. Attenuation artifact during myocardial SPECT imaging secondary to saline and silicone breast implants. Am Heart Hosp J 2007; 5(3):195–196

Santana C, Candel J, Castell J, Aguadé S, García A, Canela T, González JM, Cortadellas J, Ortega D, Soler J. Diagnostic accuracy of technetium-99m- MIBI myocardial SPECT in women and men. J Nucl Med 1998; 39:751–755

Normal Muga Study

Meinardi MT, van Veldhuisen DJ, Gietema JA, Dolsma WV, Boomsma F, van den Berg MP, Volkers C, Haaksma J, de Vries

EG, Sleijfer DT, van der Graaf WT. Prospective evaluation of early cardiac damage induced by epirubicin-containing adjuvant chemotherapy and locoregional radiotherapy in breast cancer patients. J Clin Oncol 2001; 19(10):2746–2753

Singhal PK, Ilikovic N. Doxorubicin-induced cardiomyopathy. N Engl J Med 1998; 339:900–905

Skrypniuk J, Bailey D, Cosgriff P, Fleming J, Houston A, Jarrit P, Whalley D. UK audit of left ventricular ejection fraction eestimation from equilibrium ECG gated blood poll images. Nucl Med Commun 2005; 26:205–215

Left Bundle-Branch Block (LBBB)

Burns RJ, Galligan L, Wright LM. Lawans S, Burke RJ, Gladstone PJ. Improved specificity of myocardial thallium-201 single-photon emission computed tomography in patients with left bundle branch block by dipyridamole. Am J Cardiol 1991; 68:504–508

Jukema JW, Van der Wall EE, Vis-Melsen MJ, Kruyswijk, Bruschke AV. Dypiridamole thallium-201 scintigraphy for improved detection of left anterior descending coronary artery stenosis in patients with left bundle branch block. Eur Heart J 1993; 14:53–56

Larcos G, Brown M, Gibbons R. Role of dipyridamole thallium-201 imaging in left bundle branch block. Am J Cardiol 1991; 68:1097–1098

Mahrholdt H, Zhydkov A, Hager S, Meinhard G, Wagner A, Sechtem U. Left ventricular wall motion abnormalities as well as reduced wall thickness can cause false positive results of routine SPECT perfusion imaging for detection of myocardial infarction. Eur Heart J 2005; 26:2127–2135

Ono S, Nohara R, Kambara H, Okuda K, Kawai C. Regional myocardial perfusion and glucosa metabolism in experimental left bundle Branco block. Circulation 1992; 85:1125–1131

Skalidis EI, Vardas PE. Guidelines on the management of stable angina pectoris. Eur Heart J 2006; 27:2606–2616

Travin MI, Flores AR, Boucher CA, Newell BA, La Raia PJ. Silent versus symptomatic ischaemia during a thallium-201 exercise test. Am J Cardiol 1991; 68:1600–1608

Wagdy H, Hodge D, Christian T, Miller T, Gibbons R. Pronostic value of vasodilator myocardial perfusion imaging in patients with left bundle branch block. Circulation 1998; 97: 1563–1570

Ischemia in Ada Territory

Hambye AS, Vervaet A, Dobbeleir A. Variability of left ventricular ejection fraction and volumes with quantitative gated SPECT: influence of algorithm, pixel size and reconstruction parameters in small and normal-sized hearts. Eur J Nucl Med Mol Imaging 2004; 31:1606–1613

Santana CA, Garcia EV, Vansant JP, Krawczynska EG, Folks RD, Cooke CD, Faber TL. Gated stress-only 99mTc myocardial perfusion SPECT imaging accurately assesses coronary artery disease. Nucl Med Commun 2003; 24:241–249

Ischemia in the Right Coronary Artery Territory

Castell Conesa J, Santana Boado C, Candell Riera J, Aguadé Bruix S, Olona M, Canela T et al Stress myocardial gammatomography in the diagnosis of multivessel coronary disease. Rev Esp Cardiol 1997; 50:635–642

Van Train KF, Areeda J, Garcia EV, Cooke CD, Maddahi J, Kiat H et al Quantitative same-day rest-stress technetium-99m-sestamibi SPECT: definition and validation of stress normal limits and criteria for abnormality. J Nucl Med 1993; 34: 1494–1502

Van Train KF, Garcia EV, Maddahi J, Areeda J, Cooke CD, Kiat H et al Multicenter trial validation for quantitative analysis of same-day rest-stress technetium-99m-sestamibi myocardial tomograms. J Nucl Med 1994; 35:609–618

Inducible Ischemia in the Cx Territory

Haraldsson H, Ohlsson M, Edenbrandt L. Value of exercise data for the interpretation of myocardial perfusion SPECT. J Nucl Cardiol 2002; 9:169–173

Steele P, Sklar J, Kirch D, Vogel R, Rhodes CA. Thallium-201 myocardial imaging during maximal and submaximal exercise: comparison of submaximal exercise with propranolol. Am Heart J 1983; 106:1353–1357

Non Transmural Infarct

Burak Z, Akin H, Buket S, Sagcan A, Argon M, Atay Y et al The role of 99Tcm-tetrofosmin myocardial perfusion scintigraphy in the assessment of patients with previous myocardial infarction: a comparative study with 201Tl. Nucl Med Commun 1998; 19(2):127–136

Kula M, Tutus A, Abaci A, Oguzhan A, Arslan SM, Ergin A. Comparison between rest technetium-99m-tetrofosmin and rest-redistribution thallium-201 SPECT in stable patients with healed myocardial infarction. Nucl Med Commun 2001; 22(12):1317–1324

Infarct in Apex and Antero-Infero Apical Segments Without Residual Ischemia. Inducible Ischemia in Infero-Lateral Side

Burns RJ, Gibbons RJ, Yi Q, Roberts RS, Miller TD, Schaer GL et al The relationships of left ventricular ejection fraction, end-systolic volume index and infarct size to six-month mortality after hospital discharge following myocardial infarction treated by thrombolysis. J Am Coll Cardiol 2002; 39(1): 30–36

Gjertsson P, Lomsky M, Richter J, Ohlsson M, Tout D, van Aswegen A et al The added value of ECG-gating for the diagnosis of myocardial infarction using myocardial perfusion scintigraphy and artificial neural networks. Clin Physiol Funct Imaging 2006; 26(5):301–304

Extensive Infarct Without Residual Ischemia

Elhendy A, Schinkel AF, van Domburg RT, Bax JJ, Valkema R, Poldermans D. Prognostic value of stress Tc-99m tetrofosmin SPECT in patients with previous myocardial infarction: impact of scintigraphic extent of coronary artery disease. J Nucl Cardiol 2004; 11(6):704–709

Miller TD, Christian TF, Hopfenspirger MR, Hodge DO, Gersh BJ, Gibbons RJ. Infarct size after acute myocardial infarction measured by quantitative tomographic 99mTc sestamibi imaging predicts subsequent mortality. Circulation 1995; 92(3): 334–341

Infarct With Residual Ischemia

Hachamovitch R, Berman DS, Shaw LJ, Kiat H, Cohen I, Cabico JA et al Incremental prognostic value of myocardial perfusion single photon emission computed tomography for the prediction of cardiac death: differential stratification for risk of cardiac death and myocardial infarction. Circulation 1998; 97(6):535–543

Kroll D, Farah W, McKendall GR, Reinert SE, Johnson LL. Prognostic value of stress-gated Tc-99m sestamibi SPECT after acute myocardial infarction. Am J Cardiol 2001; 87(4): 381–386

Sharir T, Germano G, Kavanagh PB, Lai S, Cohen I, Lewin HC Zellweger MJ, Berman DS et al Incremental prognostic value of post-stress left ventricular ejection fraction and volume by gated myocardial perfusion single photon emission computed tomography. Circulation 1999; 100(10):1035–1042

Multivessel Disease

Candell J, Aguadé S. Seguimiento y valoración pronóstica de la cardiopatía isquémica estable. In: Candell J, Castell J, Aguadé S (eds) Cardiología Nuclear en la Práctica Clínica. Aula Médica Ediciones, Madrid, 2003

Elhendy A, Sozzi FB, van Domburg RT, Bax JJ, Geleijnse ML, Valkema R, Krenning EP, Roelandt JR. Accuracy of exercise stress technetium 99m sestamibi SPECT imaging in the evaluation of the extent and location of coronary artery disease in patients with an earlier myocardial infarction. J Nucl Cardiol 2000; 7:432–438

Giubbini R, Campini R, Milan E, Zoccarato O, Orlandi C, Rossini P, Giannuzzi P, La Canna G, Galli M.. Evaluation of technetium-99m-sestamibi lung uptake: correlation with left ventricular function. J Nucl Med 1995; 36:58–63

Iskandrian AS, Heo J, Lemlek J, Ogilby JD, Untereker WJ, Iskandrian B, Cave V. Identification of high-risk patients with left main and three-vessel coronary artery disease by adenosine-single photon emission computed tomographic thallium imaging. Am Heart J 1993; 125:1130–1135

Sharif T, Bacher-Stier C, Dhar S et al Identification of severe and extensive coronary artery disease by postexercise regional wall motion abnormalities in 99mTc sestamibi gated single-photon emission computed tomography. Am J Cardiol 2000; 86:1171–1175

Tsou SS, Sun SS, Kao A, Lin CC, Lee CC. Exercise and rest technetium-99m-tetrofosmin lung uptake: correlation with left ventricular ejection fraction in patients with coronary artery disease. Jpn Heart J 2002; 43:515–522

Myocardial Stunning

Bolli R. Myocardial 'stunning' in man. Circulation 1992; 86: 1671–1691

Kakhki VD, Zakavi SR, Sadeghi R, Yousefi A. Importance of gated imaging in both phases of myocardial perfusion SPECT: myocardial stunning after dipyridamole infusion. J Nucl Med Technol 2006; 34:88–91

Mazzadi AN, André-Fouët X, Costes N, Croisille P, Revel D, Janier MF. Mechanisms leading to reversible mechanical dysfunction in severe CAD: alternatives to myocardial stunning. Am J Physiol Heart Circ Physiol 2006; 291:H2570–H2582

Wiggers H, Nielsen SS, Holdgaard P, Flø C, Nørrelund H, Halbirk M et al Adaptation of nonrevascularized human hibernating and chronically stunned myocardium to long-term chronic myocardial ischemia. Am J Cardiol 2006; 15:1574–1580

Myocardial Viability

Altehoefer C, Kaiser HJ, Dörr R, Feinendegen C, Beilin I, Uebis R et al Fluorine-18 deoxyglucose PET for assessment of viable myocardium in perfusion defects in 99mTc-MIBI SPET: a comparative study in patients with coronary artery disease. Eur J Nucl Med 1992; 19:334–342

Candell-Riera J, Castell-Conesa J, González JM, Rosselló-Urgell J. Efficacy of stress-rest myocardial SPET with 99mTc-MIBI in predicting recovery of postrevascularization contractile function. Results of the Spanish multicenter protocol. Working Group of Nuclear Cardiology. Rev Esp Cardiol 2000; 53:903–10

Cuocolo A, Pace L, Ricciardelli B, Chiariello M, Trimarco B, Salvatore M. Identification of viable myocardium in patients with chronic coronary artery disease: comparison of thallium-201 scintigraphy with reinjection and technetium-99m-methoxyisobutyl isonitrile. J Nucl Med 1992; 33:505–511

Dakik HA, Howell JF, Lawrie GM, Espada R, Weilbaecher DG, He ZX et al Assessment of myocardial viability with 99mTc-sestamibi tomography before coronary bypass graft surgery: correlation with histopathology and postoperative improvement in cardiac function. Circulation 1997; 96: 2892–2898

Shehata AR, Mitchell J, Heller GV. Use of gated SPECT imaging in the prediction of myocardial viability. J Nucl Cardiol 1997; 4:99–100

Myocarditis

Flotats A, Carrió I. Non-invasive in vivo imaging of myocardial apoptosis and necrosis. Eur J Nucl Med Mol Imaging 2003; 30:615–630

Noriega F, Costa MI, Vilar M, Fernández R, Martín A, Lago A. Acute myocarditis. varicella virus. Rev Esp Cardiol 1998;51: 677–679

Yamaguchi T, Yasumura Y, Nakatani S, Nagaya N, Ishibashi-Ueda H, Inubushi M et al Dual SPECT imaging of Löffler's endomyocarditis in the acute phase. Circulation 2000; 102: 2019–2020

Prognostic Evaluation in Coronary Artery Disease

Ladenheim ML, Pollock BH, Rozanski A, Berman DS, Staniloff HM, Forrester JS et al Extent and severity of myocardial hypoperfusion as predictors of prognosis in patients with suspected coronary artery disease. J Am Coll Cardiol 1986; 7:464–471

Platts EA, North TL, Pickett RD, Kelly JD. Mechanism of uptake of technetium-tetrofosmin. I: uptake into isolated adult rat ventricular myocytes and subcellular localization. J Nucl Cardiol 1995; 2:317–326

Younès A, Songadele JA, Maublant J, Platts E, Pickett R, Veyre A. Mechanism of uptake of technetium-tetrofosmin. II: uptake into isolated adult rat heart mitochondria. J Nucl Cardiol 1995; 2:327–333

Chagas' Heart Disease

Marín-Nieto JA, Simoñes MV, Ayres-Nieto EM, Atrab-Santos JL, Gallo L, Amorím DS, Mariel BC.Studies of the coronary circulation in chagas' heart disease. Sao Paulo Med J 1995; 113 (2):826–834; review

Prata A. Clinical and epidemiological aspect of Chagas disease. Lancet Infect Dis 2001; 1:92–100

Punukollu G, Gowuda RM, Khan IA. Early twentieth century descriptions of Chagas heart disease. Int J Cardiol 2004; 95:347–349

Punukollu G, Gowda RM, Khan IA, Navarro VS, Vasavada BC. Clinical aspects of the Chagas' heart disease. Int J Cardiol 2007; 115:279–283

Printing and Binding: Stürtz GmbH, Würzburg